BETTER NEVE

MW00624037

Most people believe that they \
harmed by being brought intc

reflect on whether they should bring others into existence — rather than having children without even thinking about whether they should — they presume that they do them no harm. *Better Never to Have Been* challenges these assumptions. David Benatar argues that coming into existence is always a serious harm. Although the good things in one's life make one's life go better than it otherwise would have gone, one could not have been deprived by their absence if one had not existed. Those who never exist cannot be deprived. However, by coming into existence one does suffer quite serious harms that could not have befallen one had one not come into existence. Drawing on the relevant psychological literature, the author shows that there are a number of well-documented features of human psychology that explain why people systematically overestimate the quality of their lives and why they are thus resistant to the suggestion that they were seriously harmed by being brought into existence. The author then argues for the 'anti-natal' view — that it is always wrong to have children — and he shows that combining the anti-natal view with common pro-choice views about foetal moral status yield a 'pro-death' view about abortion (at the earlier stages of gestation). Anti-natalism also implies that it would be better if humanity became extinct. Although counter-intuitive for many, that implication is defended, not least by showing that it solves many conundrums of moral theory about population.

David Benatar is Professor of Philosophy at the University of Cape Town.

BETTER NEVER TO HAVE BEEN

The Harm of Coming into Existence

DAVID BENATAR

CLARENDON PRESS · OXFORD

OXFORD

UNIVERSITY PRESS

Great Clarendon Street, Oxford OX2 6DP
United Kingdom

Oxford University Press is a department of the University of Oxford.
It furthers the University's objective of excellence in research, scholarship,
and education by publishing worldwide. Oxford is a registered trade mark of
Oxford University Press in the UK and in certain other countries

© David Benatar 2006

The moral rights of the author have been asserted

First published 2006
First published in paperback 2008
Reprinted 2009, 2013

All rights reserved. No part of this publication may be reproduced, stored in
a retrieval system, or transmitted, in any form or by any means, without the
prior permission in writing of Oxford University Press, or as expressly permitted
by law, by licence or under terms agreed with the appropriate reprographics
rights organization. Enquiries concerning reproduction outside the scope of the
above should be sent to the Rights Department, Oxford University Press, at the
address above

You must not circulate this work in any other form
and you must impose this same condition on any acquirer

British Library Cataloguing in Publication Data
Data available

Library of Congress Cataloging in Publication Data
Data available

ISBN 978-0-19-954926-9

To my parents,
even though they brought me into existence;

and to my brothers,
each of whose existence, although a harm to him,
is a great benefit to the rest of us.

Preface

Each one of us was harmed by being brought into existence. That harm is not negligible, because the quality of even the best lives is very bad—and considerably worse than most people recognize it to be. Although it is obviously too late to prevent our own existence, it is not too late to prevent the existence of future possible people. Creating new people is thus morally problematic. In this book I argue for these claims and show why the usual responses to them—incredulity, if not indignation—are defective.

Given the deep resistance to the views I shall be defending, I have no expectation that this book or its arguments will have any impact on baby-making. Procreation will continue undeterred, causing a vast amount of harm. I have written this book, then, not under the illusion that it will make (much) difference to the number of people there will be but rather from the opinion that what I have to say needs to be said whether or not it is accepted.

Many readers will be inclined to dismiss my arguments and will do so too hastily. When rejecting an unpopular view, it is extraordinarily easy to be overly confident in the force of one's responses. This is partly because there is less felt need to justify one's views when one is defending an orthodoxy. It is also partly because counter-responses from those critical of this orthodoxy, given their rarity, are harder to anticipate.

The argument I advance in this book has been enhanced as a result of a number of engaging critical responses to earlier versions. Anonymous reviewers for the *American Philosophical Quarterly* offered worthy challenges, forcing me to improve the earliest versions. The two papers I published in that journal provided the basis for Chapter 2 of this book and I am grateful for permission to use that earlier material. Those papers were considerably reworked and developed partly as a result of many comments received in the intervening years and especially while I was writing this book. I am grateful to the University of Cape Town for a sabbatical semester in 2004, during which four of the book's chapters were written. I presented material from various chapters in a number of fora, including the Philosophy Department at the University of Cape Town, Rhodes University in Grahamstown, South Africa, the Seventh World Congress of Bioethics in Sydney, Australia, and in the United States at the Jean Beer Blumenfeld Center for Ethics at Georgia State University, the Center for Bioethics at the University of Minnesota, and the Philosophy Department at the University of Alabama at Birmingham. I am grateful for the lively discussion on these occasions. For their helpful comments and suggestions, I should like to thank, among others, Andy Altman, Dan Brock, Bengt Brülde, Nick Fotion, Stephen Nathanson, Marty Perlmutter, Robert Segall, David Weberman, Bernhard Weiss, and Kit Wellman.

I am most grateful to the two reviewers for Oxford University Press, David Wasserman and David Boonin. They gave extensive comments that helped me anticipate the kinds of responses critical readers of the published work could have. I have attempted to raise and reply to these in revising the manuscript. I am sure that the book is much better for having considered their objections, even if they are not convinced by my replies. I am acutely aware, however, that there is always room for improvement and I only wish that I knew now, rather than later (or never), what improvements could be made.

Finally, I should like to thank my parents and brothers for all they do and for all they are. This book is dedicated to them.

DB

Cape Town
8 December 2005

Contents

I

Introduction

Life is so terrible, it would have been better not to have been born. Who is so lucky? Not one in a hundred thousand!

Jewish saying

The central idea of this book is that coming into existence is always a serious harm. That idea will be defended at length, but the basic insight is quite simple: Although the good things in one's life make it go better than it otherwise would have gone, one could not have been deprived by their absence if one had not existed. Those who never exist cannot be deprived. However, by coming into existence one does suffer quite serious harms that could not have befallen one had one not come into existence.

To say that the basic insight is quite simple is not to say that either it or what we can deduce from it will be undisputed. I shall consider all the anticipated objections in due course, and shall argue that they fail. The implication of all this is that coming into existence, far from ever constituting a net benefit, always constitutes a net harm. Most people, under the influence of powerful biological dispositions towards optimism, find this conclusion intolerable. They are still more indignant at the further implication that we should not create new people.

Creating new people, by having babies, is so much a part of human life that it is rarely thought even to require a justification. Indeed, most people do not even think about whether they should or should not make a baby. They just make one. In other words, procreation is usually the consequence of sex rather than the result of a decision to bring people into existence. Those who do indeed *decide* to have a child might do so for any number of reasons, but among these reasons cannot be the interests of the potential child. One can never have a child for that child's sake. That much should be apparent to everybody, even those who reject the stronger view for which I argue in this book—that not only does one not benefit people by bringing them into existence, but one *always* harms them.[1]

My argument applies not only to humans but also to all other sentient beings. Such beings do not simply exist. They exist in a way that there is something that it feels like to exist. In other words, they are not merely objects but also subjects. Although sentience is a later evolutionary development and is a more complex state of being than insentience, it is far from clear that it is a better state of being. This is because sentient existence comes at a significant cost. In being able to experience, sentient beings are able to, and do, experience *unpleasantness*.

Although I think that coming into existence harms all sentient beings and I shall sometimes speak about all such beings, my focus will be on humans. There are a few reasons for this focus, other than the sheer convenience of it. The first is that people find the conclusion hardest to accept when it applies to themselves. The focus on humans, rather than on all sentient life, reinforces its application to humans. A second reason is that, with one exception, the argument has most practical significance when applied to humans because we can act on it by desisting from producing children. The exception is the case of human breeding of animals,[1]

---

[1] I treat this as an *exception* because humans breed only a small proportion of all species of sentient animals. Although this is an exceptional case, it has great

from which we could also desist. A third reason for focusing on humans is that those humans who do not desist from producing children cause suffering to those about whom they tend to care most—their own children. This may make the issues more vivid for them than they otherwise would be.

WHO IS SO LUCKY?

A version of the view I defend in this book is the subject of some humour:

Life is so terrible, it would have been better not to have been born. Who is so lucky? Not one in a hundred thousand![2]

Sigmund Freud describes this quip as a 'nonsensical joke',[3] which raises the question whether my view is similarly nonsensical. Is it

---

significance, given the amount of harm inflicted on those animals that humans breed for food and other commodities, and is thus worthy of brief discussion now. One particularly poor argument in defence of eating meat is that if humans did not eat animals, those animals would not have been brought into existence in the first place. Humans would simply not have bred them in the numbers they do breed them. The claim is that although these animals are killed, this cost to them is outweighed by the benefit to them of having been brought into existence. This is an appalling argument for many reasons (some of which are outlined by Robert Nozick. See his *Anarchy, State and Utopia* (Oxford: Blackwell, 1974) 38–9). First, the lives of many of these animals are so bad that even if one rejected my argument one would still have to think that *they* were harmed by being brought into existence. Secondly, those who advance this argument fail to see that it could apply as readily to human babies that are produced only to be eaten. Here we see quite clearly that being brought into existence only to be killed for food is no benefit. It is only because killing animals is thought to be acceptable that the argument is thought to have any force. In fact it adds nothing to the (mistaken) view that killing animals for food is acceptable. Finally, the argument that animals are benefited by being brought into existence only to be killed ignores the argument that I shall develop in Chapters 2 and 3—that coming into existence is itself, quite independently of how *much* the animal then suffers, always a serious harm.

[2] In the philosophical literature this Jewish witticism has been cited by Robert Nozick (*Anarchy, State and Utopia*, 337 n. 8), and Bernard Williams ('The Makropulos Case: Reflections on the Tedium of Immortality' in *Problems of the Self* (Cambridge: Cambridge University Press, 1973) 87).

[3] Freud, Sigmund, *The Standard Edition of the Complete Psychological Works of Sigmund Freud*, vii, trans. James Strachey (London: The Hogarth Press, 1960) 57.

sheer drivel to say that coming into existence is a harm and thus that it is better never to come into existence? Many people think that it is. Much of the argument in Chapter 2 will show that they are mistaken. But first some ground must be cleared of confusion.

Dr Freud says that anybody 'who is not born is not a mortal man at all, and there is no good and no best for him'.[4] Here Dr Freud anticipates an aspect of what is called the 'non-identity' problem, which I shall discuss at length in Chapter 2. Some contemporary philosophers offer a similar objection when they deny that one could be better off not being born. The never-existent cannot be benefited and cannot be better off.

I shall not claim that the never-existent literally are better off. Instead, I shall argue that coming into existence is always bad for those who come into existence. In other words, although we may not be able to say of the never-existent that never existing is good for them, we can say of the existent that existence is bad for them. There is no absurdity here, or so I shall argue.

Once we acknowledge that coming into existence can be a harm, we might then want to speak loosely about never coming into existence being 'better'. This is not to say that it is better for the never-existent, nor that the never-existent are benefited. I grant that there is even something odd about speaking about the 'never-existent', because that is surely a referentless term. There clearly are not any never-existent people. It is, however, a convenient

[4] Ibid. Although this is the deepest concern Dr Freud has with the quip, he has others too. These, however, arise from his version of the quip, which sounds particularly nonsensical. He says: 'Never to be born would be the best thing for mortal men.' 'But', adds the philosophical comment in *Fliegende Blätter*, 'this happens to scarcely one person in a hundred thousand.' (Ibid.) The embellishment that never being born 'happens to *scarcely* one in a hundred thousand' does add to the joke's incongruity. Never being born happens to not one in a hundred thousand, and not to *scarcely* one in a hundred thousand. (James Strachey describes the *Fliegende Blätter* as a 'well-known comic weekly'. I leave to others the minor, but interesting, historical question whether the *Fliegende Blätter* drew on Jewish wit or whether it was the source of this particular piece of Jewish humour, or whether both draw on some other source.)

term, of which we can make some sense. By it we mean those possible people who never become actual.

With this in mind, consider the joke again. It can be viewed as making two claims: (1) that it is better not to be born, and (2) that nobody is lucky enough not to be born. We now see that there *is* a (loose) sense in which one can say that it is better not to be born. It is an indirect way of saying that coming into existence is always a harm. And there is nothing nonsensical in claiming that *nobody* is lucky enough never to have come into existence, even though it would have been (playful) nonsense to claim that there are some people who *are* lucky enough not to come into existence.

In any event, the fact that one can construct a joke about the view that coming into existence is always a harm, does not show that that view itself is laughable nonsense. Although we can laugh at silliness we can also laugh about very serious matters. It is into the latter category that I place jokes about the harm of coming into existence.[5] Lest it be thought that the arguments I advance are intended as mere philosophical games or jokes, I should emphasize that I am entirely serious in my arguments and I believe the conclusions.

I am serious about these matters because what lies in the balance is the presence or absence of vast amounts of harm. I shall show in Chapter 3 that each life contains a great deal of bad—much more than people usually think. The only way to guarantee that some future possible person will not suffer this harm is to ensure that that possible person never becomes an actual person. Not only is this harm all readily avoidable, but it is also so utterly pointless (at least if we consider only the interests of the potential person and not also the interests others might have in that person's coming

[5] There are other such jokes. For example, it has been joked that life is a sexually transmitted terminal disease. (In cases of artificial reproduction, life is not sexually transmitted, but it remains a terminal disease.) Others have jested that we are born cold, naked, hungry, and wet—and that it is downhill from there. (Although neonates cry not from a recognition of this, their cries, on my view, are ironically appropriate.)

into existence). As I shall show in Chapter 2, the positive features of life, although good for those who exist, cannot justify the negative features that accompany them. Their absence would not have been a deprivation for one who never came into existence.

It is curious that while good people go to great lengths to spare their children from suffering, few of them seem to notice that the one (and only) guaranteed way to prevent all the suffering of their children is not to bring those children into existence in the first place.[6] There are many reasons why people do not notice this, or why, if they do notice it, that they do not act on the realization, but the interests of the potential children cannot be among them, as I shall argue.

Nor is the harm produced by the creation of a child usually restricted to that child. The child soon finds itself motivated to procreate, producing children who, in turn, develop the same desire. Thus any pair of procreators can view themselves as occupying the tip of a generational iceberg of suffering.[7] They experience the bad in their own lives. In the ordinary course of events they will experience only some of the bad in their children's and possibly grandchildren's lives (because these offspring usually survive their progenitors), but beneath the surface of the current generations lurk increasingly larger numbers of descendents and their misfortunes. Assuming that each couple has three children, an original pair's cumulative descendents over ten generations amount to 88,572 people. That constitutes a lot of pointless,

[6] Rivka Weinberg makes a similar point when she says that 'many of the parents who are willing to make huge sacrifices for the sake of their desperately ill children may never consider that the most important sacrifice they ought to make is not to create these desperately ill children in the first place.' ('Procreative Justice: A Contractualist Account', *Public Affairs Quarterly*, 16/4 (2002) 406.) Her point is more restricted than mine because she applies it only to desperately ill children whereas I would apply it to all children.

[7] I owe the image of the iceberg to University of Cape Town geneticist Raj Ramesar. He uses it to represent the relationship between carriers of a genetic disorder and their (potential or actual) offspring. I have broadened the image to apply not only to those with genetic disorders but to all those (members of sentient species) with genes.

avoidable suffering. To be sure, full responsibility for it all does not lie with the original couple because each new generation faces the choice of whether to continue that line of descendents. Nevertheless, they bear some responsibility for the generations that ensue. If one does not desist from having children, one can hardly expect one's descendents to do so.

Although, as we have seen, *nobody* is lucky enough not to be born, *everybody* is *unlucky* enough to have been born—and particularly bad *luck* it is, as I shall now explain. On the quite plausible assumption that one's genetic origin is a necessary (but not sufficient) condition for having come into existence,[8] one could not have been formed by anything other than the particular gametes that produced the zygote from which one developed. This implies, in turn, that one could not have had any genetic parents other than those that one does have. It follows from this that any person's chances of having come into existence are extremely remote. The existence of any one person is dependent not only on that person's parents themselves having come into existence and having met[9] but also on their having conceived that person at the time that they did.[10] Indeed, mere moments might make a difference to which particular sperm is instrumental in a conception. The recognition of how unlikely it was that one would have come into existence, combined with the recognition that coming into existence is always a serious harm, yields the conclusion that one's having come into existence is *really* bad luck. It is bad enough when one suffers some harm. It is worse still when the chances of having been harmed are very remote.

---

[8] Derek Parfit calls this the 'Origin View'. *Reasons and Persons* (Oxford: Clarendon Press, 1984) 352.

[9] Derek Parfit asks 'how many of us could truly claim "Even if railways and motor cars had never been invented, I would still have been born"?', *Reasons and Persons*, 361.

[10] Think of how many people are conceived because of a power failure, a nocturnal noise waking their parents, or any other such opportunity merging with urge.

Now there is something misleading about this observation. This is because of all the trillions of possible people who could have come into existence and assessed the odds, *every* one of those who is in a position to assess the odds is unlucky whereas there exists *nobody* whom the odds favoured. One hundred per cent of assessors are unlucky, and nought per cent are lucky. In other words, given procreation there was an excellent chance that *somebody* would be harmed, and although the chances of any person coming into existence are small, the chances of any existing person having been harmed are one hundred per cent.

ANTI-NATALISM AND THE PRO-NATAL BIAS

I shall argue that one implication of the view that coming into existence is always a serious harm is that we should not have children. Some anti-natalist positions are founded on either a dislike of children[11] or on the interests of adults who have greater freedom and resources if they do not have and rear children.[12] My anti-natalist view is different. It arises, not from a dislike of children, but instead from a concern to avoid the suffering of potential children and the adults they would become, even if not having those children runs counter to the interests of those who would have them.

Anti-natalist views, whatever their source, run up against an extremely powerful pro-natalist bias. This bias has its roots in the evolutionary origins of human (and more primitive animal) psychology and biology. Those with pro-natal views are more likely to pass on their genes. It is part of the pro-natal bias that most

[11] W.C. Fields said that he did not like children . . . unless they were very well cooked. (Or was it that he only liked them fried?) See also Ogden Nash's poems, 'Did someone say "babies"?' and 'To a small boy standing on my shoes while I am wearing them' in *Family Reunion* (London: J. M. Dent & Sons Ltd, 1951) 5–7.

[12] Andrew Hacker refers to some of these arguments. See his review, 'The Case Against Kids', *The New York Review of Books*, 47/19 (2000) 12–18.

people simply assume that passing on one's genes is both good and a sign of superiority. With different moral views, however, survival, either of the self or of one's genes, might not be seen as an indication of being better.

The pro-natal bias manifests itself in many ways. For example, there is the assumption that one should (get married or simply cohabit in order to) produce children, and that, infertility aside, one is either backward or selfish if one does not.[13] The assumption of 'backwardness' draws on an ontogenetic or individual developmental paradigm—children do not have children, but adults do. Thus if one has not (yet) started breeding, one is not fully adult. But it is far from clear that this is the appropriate paradigm. First, knowing when *not* to have a baby and having the self-control to follow through with this is a sign of maturity not immaturity. There are all too many (pubescent) children who are having children without being adequately prepared to rear them. Second, is a related point: from a phylogenetic perspective, the impulse to procreation is extremely primitive. If 'backward' is understood as 'primitive' it is procreation that is backward, and rationally motivated non-procreation that is evolutionarily more recent and advanced.

Although non-procreation is sometimes, as I indicated above, motivated by selfish concerns, it need not be. Where people refrain from procreating in order to avoid inflicting the harm of coming into existence, their motives are altruistic not selfish. Moreover, any self-consciously altruistic motivation to have children is thoroughly misguided where the intended beneficiaries are the children, and, as I shall argue, inappropriate where they are other people or the state.

In some communities there is considerable peer and other social pressure to produce babies, and sometimes even as many

[13] Sometimes the presumption is betrayed by the word 'yet' as in 'Have you had children *yet*?' This assumption does not usually extend to (both male and female) homosexuals who do not have children, although homosexuals, whether or not they have children, are often the victims of a more vicious opprobrium. They are often regarded as perverted or disgusting rather than backward or selfish.

babies as possible. This can occur even when parents are unable to take adequate care of the large number of children they are producing.[14]

Nor are the pressures always informal. Governments not infrequently intervene, particularly, but not only, when birth rates decline, in order to encourage baby-making. This is true even where the baseline population is already high and the concern is only about birth rates falling beneath that of replacement. Here the concern is that there will be fewer people of working age and thus fewer taxpayers to support a larger ageing population.[15] For example, in Japan there were concerns that the birth rate of 1.33 children would reduce the population of 127 million people to 101 million in 2050 and 64 million by 2100.[16] The Japanese government took action. They launched the 'Plus One Plan', aimed at persuading married couples to have one extra child, and established the 'Anti Low Birthrate Measures Promotion' headquarters to coordinate the plan. One of the proposals in the plan was a ¥3.1 billion matchmaking budget to be spent on 'publicly-funded parties, boat cruises, and hiking trips for single men and women'.[17] The government also pledged financial support for couples seeking expensive fertility treatment. The 'Plus One Plan' also had provision for diverting resources to provide education loans to put children through school. Singapore developed plans to persuade citizens to produce more children. In addition to propaganda, it introduced financial incentives to have a third child, paid maternity leave, and state-funded childcare

[14] Beyer, Lisa, 'Be Fruitful and Multiply: Criticism of the ultra-Orthodox fashion for large families is coming from inside the community', *Time*, 25 October 1999, 34.

[15] I shall say more in Chapter 7 about the costs to existing people of a decreased birth rate. In the specific case of Japan, to which I shall now refer, not everybody agrees that the population decline will impact very adversely on Japanese society. See, for example, 'The incredible shrinking country', *The Economist*, 13 November 2004, 45–6.

[16] Watts, Jonathan, 'Japan opens dating agency to improve birth rate', *The Lancet*, 360 (2002) 1755.

[17] Ibid.

centres.[18] And Australia has announced a $13.3 billion 'family package' to be distributed over five years. According to that country's treasurer, if 'you can have children, it's a good thing to do'. In addition to having one child for the husband and one for the wife, he urged Australians also to have one for their country.[19]

It is well known that totalitarian regimes often encourage people, if not coerce or force them into baby-making for military reasons—given the desire for new, plentiful generations of soldiers. Crudely put, this is pro-natalism for cannon fodder. Democracies, particularly those not involved in protracted conflict, are not and need not be so crude, but this, as we have seen, does not mean that they are devoid of pro-natalism.

Even where democracies take no formal steps to increase the birth rate, we should note that democracy has an inherent bias towards pro-natalism. Given that the majority prevails (even if within certain liberal constraints), each sector of a democracy's population is incentivized to produce extra offspring in order for its interests and agendas either to prevail or at least to hold their own. Notice, by extension, that in a democracy those committed to non-procreation could never, in the long run, prevail politically against those committed to procreation.

Moreover, it is curious how democracy favours breeding over immigration. Offspring have a presumed right to citizenship, while potential immigrants do not. Imagine a polarized state consisting of two opposing ethnic groups. One increases its size by breeding and the other by immigration. Depending on who holds power, the group that grows by immigration will either be prevented from growing or it will be accused of colonialism.[20] But why should democracy favour one indigenous group over another merely because one breeds rather than increases by immigration? Why

[18] Bowring, Philip, 'For Love of Country', *Time*, 11 September 2000, 58.
[19] Reuters, 'Brace yerself Sheila, it's your patriotic duty to breed', *Cape Times*, Thursday, 13 May 2004, 1.
[20] The Arab–Jewish demographic within Israel is a case in point.

should breeding be unlimited but immigration curtailed where political outcomes are equally sensitive to both ways of enhancing population? Some may seek to answer this question by arguing that a right to procreative freedom is more important than a right to immigrate. That may indeed be an accurate description of the way the law actually works, but we can question whether that is the way it *should* be. Should somebody's freedom to create a person be more inviolable than somebody else's freedom to have a friend or family member immigrate?

Another way in which pro-natalism operates, even in the moral (and not merely the political) realm is that breeders enhance their value by having children. Parents with dependents are somehow thought to count for more. If, for example, there is some scarce resource—a donor kidney perhaps—and of the two potential recipients one is a parent of young children and one is not, the parent, all things being equal, will likely be favoured. To let a parent die is not only to thwart that person's preference to be saved, but also the preferences of his or her children that their parent be saved. It is quite true, of course, that the death of the parent will harm more people, but there is nonetheless something to be said against favouring parents. Increasing one's value by having children might be like increasing one's value by taking hostages. We might find it unfair and decide not to reward it. That may make children's lives worse, but must the cost of preventing that outcome be placed on the shoulders of those who do not have children?

None of the above is to deny that there are some societies in which anti-natal policies have been adopted. The most obvious example is China, where the government introduced a one-child-per-couple policy. A few points are noteworthy, however. First, such policies are exceptional. Secondly, they are a response to massive (rather than merely moderate) overpopulation. Thirdly, they are required precisely because they are a corrective to a very powerful pro-natal bias, and thus do not constitute a refutation of the existence of such bias.

Nor do I deny that there are some non-state critics of pro-natalism. There are those, for example, who argue that one's life is better or at least no worse[21] without children and there are those who object to the discrimination against people who are either infertile[22] or 'child-free' by choice.[23] As welcome as this opposition to pro-natalism is, most of it is inspired by concern for existing people. Very rarely do we hear criticism of pro-natalism based on what procreation does to those who are brought into existence. There is one kind of exception: those who believe that the world is too horrible a place into which to bring children. Such people believe that there happens to be too much bad in the world to make procreation acceptable. That belief must be right. I disagree only in one way with those who advance it. Unlike (most of) them, I think that there could be *much* less suffering and yet procreation would remain unacceptable. On my view there is no net benefit to coming into existence and thus coming into existence is never worth its costs. I know that that view is hard to accept. I shall defend it in some detail in Chapter 2. Sound though I believe my argument to be, I cannot but hope that I am wrong.

OUTLINE OF THE BOOK

In the remainder of this introduction I shall provide an outline of the rest of the book and offer some guidelines to readers.

The second and third chapters constitute the heart of the book. In Chapter 2 I shall argue that coming into existence is always a harm. To do this, I shall show first that coming into existence

---

[21] Missner, Marshall, 'Why Have Children?', *The International Journal of Applied Philosophy*, 3/4 (1987) 1–13.

[22] May, Elaine Tyler, 'Nonmothers as Bad Mothers: Infertility and the Maternal Instinct', in Ladd-Taylor, Molly, and Umansky, Lauri, *'Bad' Mothers: The Politics of Blame in Twentieth-Century America* (New York: NYU Press, 1998) 198–219.

[23] Burkett, Elinor, *The Baby Boon: How Family-Friendly America Cheats the Childless* (New York: The Free Press, 2000).

is sometimes a harm—a claim which ordinary people would readily embrace but which must be defended against a famous philosophical challenge. The argument that coming into existence is *always* a harm can be summarized as follows: Both good and bad things happen only to those who exist. However, there is a crucial asymmetry between the good and the bad things. The absence of bad things, such as pain, is good even if there is nobody to enjoy that good, whereas the absence of good things, such as pleasure, is bad only if there is somebody who is deprived of these good things. The implication of this is that the avoidance of the bad by never existing is a real advantage over existence, whereas the loss of certain goods by not existing is not a real disadvantage over never existing.

In the third chapter I argue that even the best lives are not only much worse than people think but also very bad. To this end, I shall argue first that life's quality is not the difference between its good and bad. Determining a life's quality is a much more complicated matter. I shall then discuss three views about the quality of life—hedonistic views, desire-fulfilment views, and objective list views—and show why life is bad irrespective of which of these views one adopts. Finally, in this chapter, I shall describe the world of suffering that we inhabit and argue that this suffering is one of the costs of producing new people. The arguments in the third chapter thus provide independent grounds even for those who are not persuaded by the arguments in the second chapter to accept the claim that coming into existence is always a (serious) harm.

In the fourth chapter I shall argue that not only is there no duty to procreate but there is a (moral) duty not to procreate. This appears to conflict with a widely recognized right to procreative freedom. I shall examine this right and its possible foundations, arguing that it is best understood as a legal right and not a moral one. Thus there is no necessary conflict with a moral duty not to produce children. I then turn to the question of disability and wrongful life. I shall consider various disability rights arguments and show how my views, curiously, both lend support to these arguments against their usual opponents, but in the end undermine the views of both disability rights and their opponents. Next I shall turn to the implications of my views for assisted and artificial reproduction, before concluding with a discussion about whether producing children treats them as mere means.

In the fifth chapter, I shall show how combining typical pro-choice views about fetal moral status with my conclusions about the harm of coming into existence produces a 'pro-death' view of abortion. More specifically, I shall argue that if fetuses at the earlier stages of gestation have not yet come into existence in the morally relevant sense, and coming into existence is always a harm, it would be better if we aborted fetuses in those earlier stages. Along the way I shall distinguish four kinds of interest and ask which of these is morally significant, I shall discuss the question of when consciousness begins, and then defend my and pro-choice views about abortion against the most interesting challenges—those of Richard Hare and Don Marquis.

The sixth chapter will examine two related sets of questions: those about population and those about extinction. The population questions are questions about how many people there should be. The extinction questions are questions about whether future human extinction is to be regretted and whether it would be worse if human extinction would come earlier rather than later. My answer to the population question is that there should, ideally, be no (more) people. However, I shall consider arguments that might allow a phased extinction. In answering the extinction question, I shall suggest that although extinction may be bad for those who precede it, particularly those who immediately precede it, the state of human extinction itself is not bad. Indeed, I shall argue that it would be better, all things being equal, if human extinction happened earlier rather than later. In addition to these arguments of general interest, I shall also show how my views solve many well-known problems in moral theorizing about population size. Here the focus will be on Part Four of Derek Parfit's book, *Reasons and Persons*, showing how my views can solve the 'non-identity problem', avoid the 'absurd conclusion' and the 'mere addition problem', and explain 'asymmetry'.

In the concluding chapter I shall discuss a number of issues. I shall consider the question whether the implausibility of my conclusions counts against my arguments and I shall argue against the optimistic insistence that I must be wrong. I shall demonstrate that my arguments are not as incompatible with religious thinking as many people might think. I shall examine questions about death and suicide. More specifically, I shall argue that one can think that coming into existence is always a harm without having to think that continuing to exist is always worse than death. Thus death may be bad for us even if coming into existence is also bad. It follows that suicide is not an inevitable implication of my view, even though it may be one possible response, at least in some cases. Finally, the conclusion will show that although the anti-natal view is philanthropically motivated, there are very compelling misanthropic arguments for the same conclusion.

A READER'S GUIDE

Not every reader may be inclined or have time to read the whole book and thus I offer some advice on prioritizing. The most important chapters are Chapter 2 (and more specifically the section entitled 'Why coming into existence is always a harm') and Chapter 3. The opening section of the concluding chapter, Chapter 7, is also important for those who think that my conclusions should be rejected on the grounds of being deeply counter-intuitive.

Chapters 4, 5, and 6 all presuppose the conclusions of Chapters 2 and 3 and thus cannot be read profitably without the earlier chapters in mind. Whereas Chapter 5 does not rest on Chapter 4, Chapter 6 does presuppose the conclusions of Chapter 4 (but not of Chapter 5). This logical ordering of the chapters roughly approximates another ordering. Chapter 2 is the 'bad news', Chapter 3 the 'worse news' and one or more of Chapters 4, 5, and 6 (depending on one's views) contains the 'worst news'.

Much of this book will be readily accessible to an intelligent reader who has no background in Philosophy. There are some sections that, of necessity, are somewhat more technical. Although grasping every detail of these sections may be more difficult, the gist of the argument should nonetheless be clear. However, there are some sections that a reader less interested in the more technical details could skip. This is true of the occasional paragraph scattered throughout the book, but it is also true of more substantial sections.

In Chapter 5, the first six paragraphs of 'Four kinds of interest' are crucial to that chapter. Those readers not interested in how that taxonomy maps onto competing taxonomies in the literature of moral philosophy may skip the rest of that section.

The most technical parts of the book are in Chapter 6, in the section entitled 'Solving Problems in Moral Theory about Population'. In that section I show how my views help solve problems that have been discussed in an extensive philosophical literature about future people and optimum population size. Those without knowledge of and interest in this literature could skip that section. Doing so will make it somewhat more difficult to understand much of my discussion, later in Chapter 6, about phased extinction. Some of that discussion is also quite technical and thus could also be avoided. Any reader who does that need only know that I argue that my views might allow, under some conditions, for a phased extinction, whereby fewer and fewer children are brought into existence in each of (only) a few successive generations, rather than an immediate cessation of all baby-making.

2

Why Coming into Existence Is Always a Harm

Never to have been born is best
But if we must see the light, the next best
Is quickly returning whence we came.
When youth departs, with all its follies,
Who does not stagger under evils? Who escapes them?

Sophocles[1]

Sleep is good, death is better; but of course,
The best would be never to have been born at all.

Heinrich Heine[2]

CAN COMING INTO EXISTENCE EVER BE A HARM?

Before it can be argued that coming into existence is *always* a harm, it must first be shown that it can *ever* be a harm to come into existence. Some might wonder why this is so, for common sense

---

[1] Sophocles, *Oedipus at Colonus*, lines 1224–31.
[2] Heine, Heinrich, *Morphine*, lines 15–16.

suggests that a life *can* be so bad that coming into existence with such a life is most certainly a harm. This view, however, faces a serious challenge—one that has often been called the 'non-identity problem'[3] or the 'paradox of future individuals'.[4] I begin, then, by explaining this problem and showing how it can be resolved.

The problem arises in those cases where the only alternative to bringing a person into existence with a poor quality of life is not to bring that person into existence at all. In such circumstances it is impossible to bring the same person into existence without the condition that is thought to be harmful. This may occur, for instance, where prospective parents are carriers of a serious genetic disorder which, for one reason or another, they will pass on to their offspring. The choice is either to bring a defective child into existence or not to bring that child into existence at all.[5] On other occasions the defective condition is not attributable to the person's constitution, genetic or otherwise, but rather to his[6] environment. This is the case with the fourteen-year old girl who has a baby but because of her own tender age is unable to provide it with adequate opportunities.[7] If she conceives a child when she is older and better able to care for it, it will not be the same child (because it will have been formed from different gametes). So her alternative to bringing a socially compromised child into existence when she is fourteen years old is not to bring that child into existence at all, irrespective of whether she later has another child.

[3] Parfit, Derek, *Reasons and Persons*, 359.
[4] Kavka, Gregory S., 'The Paradox of Future Individuals' in *Philosophy and Public Affairs*, 11/2 (1982) 93–112.
[5] The development of genetic engineering may reduce the number of instances in which one is faced with such a choice, as it may be possible to bring the person into existence *and* correct the defect. However, it seems that at least some disorders will be such that eliminating them will amount to altering the identity of the being subject to the genetic engineering. In such cases the choice will be between bringing a defective child into existence or bringing a healthy, but different, child into existence.
[6] For a defence of the use of this pronoun see Benatar, David, 'Sexist Language: Alternatives to the Alternatives', *Public Affairs Quarterly*, 19/1 (2005) 1–9.
[7] The example is Derek Parfit's. See his *Reasons and Persons*, 358.

Whereas the claim that coming into existence is always a harm runs counter to most (but not all) people's intuitions, the claim that coming into existence in the aforementioned cases is a harm accords very well with popular intuition. Yet many jurists and philosophers have thought, for reasons I shall explain, that there is a logical obstacle to claiming that people whose impairments are inseparable from their existence are harmed by being brought into existence disabled.

Lives worth living and lives not worth living

There is a common distinction, in the literature about this problem, between impairments that make a life not worth living and impairments that, although severe, are not so bad as to make life not worth living. Some have made the strong claim that even where impairments make a life not worth living, we cannot claim that those people whose existence is inseparable from such impairments are harmed by being brought into existence. In support of this, the following sort of argument is advanced:

1. For something to harm somebody, it must make that person worse off.[8]
2. The 'worse off' relation is a relation between two states.
3. Thus, for somebody to be worse off in some state (such as existence), the alternative state, with which it is compared, must be one in which he is less badly (or better) off.
4. But non-existence is not a state in which anybody can be, and thus cannot be compared with existence.

[8] In this formulation, I gloss over the issue of what it must make the person worse off *than*. This is because it does not make any difference, in the context of this argument, whether we say 'worse off than he was' or 'worse off than he would have been'. For more on problems with each of these views see, Feinberg, Joel, 'Wrongful Life and the Counterfactual Element in Harming' in *Freedom and Fulfilment* (Princeton: Princeton University Press, 1992) 3–36.

5. Thus coming into existence cannot be *worse* than never coming into existence.

6. Therefore, coming into existence cannot be a harm.

One way of responding to this argument is to deny the first premiss's claim that for something to harm somebody it *must* (that is, always) make that person *worse* off. For something to harm somebody, it might be sufficient that it be *bad* for that person[9] on condition that the alternative would not have been bad.[10] On this view of harm, coming into existence can be a harm. If a life is bad for the person brought into existence, as it must be if the life is not worth living, then that person's coming into existence is a harm (given that the alternative would not have been bad).

Joel Feinberg offers a different response to the argument that coming into existence can never be a harm. Instead of denying that to harm is to make somebody worse off, he disputes the assumption that to be worse off in a particular condition, it must be the case that one would have existed in the alternative condition with which it is compared.[11] What we mean when we say that somebody would have been better off not having come into existence is that non-existence would have been preferable. Professor Feinberg offers the analogy of judgements about *ceasing* to exist. When a person claims that his life is so bad that he would be better off dead, he need not mean literally that were he to die he would exist in some better state (although some people do believe this). Instead he may

[9] Derek Parfit makes a similar move (suggested to him by Jeff McMahan), but with reference to 'better' rather than 'worse', in his argument that causing somebody to exist *could* benefit that person. Professor Parfit says that we 'may admit. . .causing someone to exist cannot be *better* for this person. But it may be *good* for this person.' (*Reasons and Persons*, 489.)

[10] This qualification avoids the complications (for a comparative view of harm) posed by those cases such as the following: You are trapped in a burning car and the only way I can save your life is by cutting off your hand and releasing you. Being handless is surely bad for you, but, all things being equal, I have nonetheless benefited you. And if I have benefited you then I have not harmed you (all things considered).

[11] Feinberg, Joel, 'Wrongful Life and the Counterfactual Element in Harming'.

mean that he prefers *not to be*, rather than to continue living in his condition. He has determined that his life is not worth living—that it is not worth continuing to be. Just as life can be so bad that ceasing to exist is preferable, so life can be so bad that never coming into existence is preferable. Comparing somebody's existence with his non-existence is not to compare two possible conditions of that person. Rather it is to compare his existence with an alternative state of affairs in which he does not exist.

It has generally been thought that those cases where the impairment, although severe, is not so bad as to make life not worth living are more difficult than cases where the impairment is so great as to make life not worth living. It has been said that because the former, by definition, are cases of lives worth living, one cannot judge never existing to be preferable to existing with such a life. The force of this argument, however, rests on a crucial ambiguity in the expression 'a life worth living'—an ambiguity I shall now probe.

Lives worth starting and lives worth continuing

The expression 'a life worth living' is ambiguous between 'a life worth continuing'—let us call this *the present-life sense*—and 'a life worth starting'—let us call this *the future-life sense*.[12] 'A life worth continuing', like 'a life not worth continuing', are judgements one can make about an already existent person. 'A life worth starting', like 'a life not worth starting', are judgements one can make about a potential but non-existent being. Now the problem is that a number of people have employed the present-life sense and applied it to future-life cases,[13] which are quite different. When

[12] A similar ambiguity characterizes the use of the expression 'a minimally decent life' in discussions of wrongful life. This expression may mean 'a life that is sufficiently decent to be worth continuing' (the present-life sense) or 'a life that is sufficiently decent to be worth bringing about' (the future-life sense).

[13] e.g. Parfit, Derek, *Reasons and Persons*, 358–9; Feinberg, Joel, 'Wrongful Life and the Counterfactual Element in Harming', 26. Bernard Williams makes the same mistake when he says 'I see no way of denying that one who resents his own

they distinguish between impairments that make a life not worth living and impairments that, though severe, are not so bad as to make life not worth living, they are making the judgements in the present-life cases. Those lives not worth living are those that would not be worth continuing. Similarly, those lives worth living are those that are worth continuing. But the problem is that these notions are then applied to future-life cases.[14] In this way, we are led to make judgements about future-life cases by the standards of present-life cases.

However, quite different standards apply in the two kinds of case. The judgement that an impairment is so bad that it makes life not worth continuing is usually made at a much higher threshold than the judgement that an impairment is sufficiently bad to make life not worth beginning. That is to say, if a life is not worth continuing, a fortiori it is not worth beginning. It does not follow, however, that if a life is worth continuing it is worth beginning or that if it is not worth beginning it would not be worth continuing. For instance, while most people think that living life without a limb does not make life so bad that it is worth ending, most (of the same) people also think that it is better not to bring into existence somebody who will lack a limb. We require stronger justification for ending a life than for not starting one.[15]

We are now in a position to understand how it might be preferable not to begin a life worth living. The paradoxical appearance

existence prefers that he should not have existed; and no way of interpreting that preference except in terms of thinking that one's life is *not worth living*.' ('Resenting one's own existence' in *Making Sense of Humanity* (Cambridge: Cambridge University Press, 1995) 228.)

[14] Joel Feinberg, for example, says the following in the context of wrongful life suits: 'Is non-existence in fact ever rationally preferable to a severely encumbered existence? Surely, in most cases of suffering and impairment we think of death as even worse.' ('Wrongful Life and the Counterfactual Element in Harming', 17.) In the context 'non-existence' refers to never existing (as opposed to ceasing to exist). Yet he answers the question by contrasting the impaired life with *death*.

[15] Something similar is true in more trivial cases. Consider, for example, an evening at the cinema. A film might be bad enough that it would have been better not to have gone to see it, but not so bad that it is worth leaving before it finishes.

of such a view rests on understanding 'a life worth living' in the future-life sense. Clearly, it would be odd to claim that it is preferable not to start a life that is worth starting. However, the future-life sense is not the relevant sense in this context, because we are considering the contrast to a life not worth continuing—namely a life worth continuing. There is nothing paradoxical about the claim that it is preferable not to begin a life that would be worth continuing.

My argument so far rests on the view that there is a morally important distinction between future-life and present-life cases. There are some lines of argument that threaten to diminish the importance of this distinction and thus weaken my case. I wish to reply to each.

First, I consider an argument of Derek Parfit's. He suggests that if I am benefited by having my life saved *just after* it started, (even if at the expense of acquiring some severe but non-catastrophic impairment), then it is not implausible to claim that I am benefited by having my life started (with such an impairment).[16] This argument seeks to minimize the significance of the distinction between future-life and present-life cases. On this view it is not unreasonable to think that impairments that are inflicted in the course of saving a life are morally comparable to similar impairments that are inseparable from bringing a life into existence.

One objection to this argument is that it rests on a shaky premise—namely, that one is benefited by having one's life saved just after it is started, if that entails one's having a severe (even though non-catastrophic) defect for the rest of one's life. Although at first sight this premise may seem firm and widely accepted, a little probing reveals its weakness. The problem is that it is

---

[16] This argument, without the parenthetical parts, can be found in 'Whether Causing Somebody To Exist Can Benefit This Person' in *Reasons and Persons*, appendix G, 489. The version of the argument that includes the parenthetical parts was suggested by Derek Parfit in comments on an early ancestor of this chapter. For these comments I am grateful.

implicitly assumed that there is some point, even if approximate, at which a being comes into existence in a morally relevant sense—that is, in the sense of having an interest deserving of moral consideration. However, as the extensive literature about abortion suggests, coming into existence in the morally relevant sense is more like a very extended process than an event. I was once a fertilized ovum. Arguably my conception[17] was the time that I came into existence in a strictly ontological sense. But it is much less clear that this was also the moment that I came into existence in a morally relevant sense. Although most people would agree that to save my life now at the cost of my leg would confer a net benefit on me, many fewer people would think that saving the life of a conceptus at the cost of its living a life without a leg constitutes a net benefit. That is why many more people support 'therapeutic' abortions even for non-catastrophic defects than condemn life-saving amputations on ordinary adults. Some people support even infanticide or at least passive euthanasia for neonates with severe but non-catastrophic disabilities even though they would not judge similar conduct to be in the interests of non-infant children and adults with such defects. Those who exist (in the morally relevant sense) have interests in existing. These interests, once fully developed, are typically very strong and thus, where there is a conflict, they override interests in not being impaired. However, where there are no (or very weak) interests in existing, causing impairments (by bringing people with defects into being) cannot be warranted by the protection of such interests. The scope of the class of beings without interests (or with very weak interests) in existing is a matter of dispute. (Does it include embryos, zygotes, infants?) In Chapter 5 I argue that at least zygotes, embryos, and

---

[17] Or by about fourteen days thereafter, once the possibility of monozygotic twinning has largely passed. One would have to date the beginning of a being's irreversible individuality still later if one wished to take the phenomenon of conjoined twins into account. (For more on this, see Singer, Peter; Kuhse, Helga; Buckle, Stephen; Dawson, Karen; and Kasimba, Pascal, eds., *Embryo Experimentation* (Cambridge: Cambridge University Press, 1990) 57–9, 66–8.)

fetuses until quite late in gestation have not begun existing in a morally relevant sense and that coming to exist in a morally relevant sense is a gradual process.

These reflections undermine the notion that there is any such stage as '*just* after one comes into existence' (in the morally relevant sense of 'comes into existence'). If we view coming into existence (in the morally relevant sense) as the extended process that it is, then we are likely to permit greater life-saving sacrifices as a being's interest in existing develops. The neat contrast between starting a life and saving a life *just after* it is started falls away. It accordingly becomes much less plausible to make an inference from the case of saving a life after it has started to the case of starting a life, as they are seen to be much farther apart.

Now some might think that the gradualist view about coming into existence undermines my distinction between future-life cases and present-life cases. This, however, is not true. That the distinction between them is a gradual one does not render the distinction void. Nothing I have said excludes the possibility of a middle ground linking the two kinds of cases. Nor is the moral significance of the distinction compromised so long as one does not, as I do not, reject a moral sensitivity to the gradualism of the continuum that links clear future-life cases with clear present-life cases.

The next possible threat to the distinction between present-life cases and future-life cases comes from a line of reasoning advanced by Joel Feinberg. He suggests, as I indicated earlier, that we understand the claim that somebody would have been better off not coming into existence as the assertion that that being's never existing would have been preferable. This assertion, he claims correctly, is not plagued by any logical difficulties. However, he goes on to advance an account of when it is preferable not to come into being,[18] such that, in almost all cases, never existing cannot be said to be preferable. He distinguishes between judgements

[18] 'Wrongful Life and the Counterfactual Element in Harming', 20–3.

by competent adults or mature older children that it would have been preferable if they had never come into existence, and similar judgements made by proxies on behalf of those who are so extremely impaired that they cannot make judgements themselves. In the case of the extremely impaired, he thinks, it is insufficient that the judgement of the preferability of never existing be *consistent with reason*. It must be *dictated* (or required) *by reason*. He thinks that this requirement is met for very few disabling conditions—those where death is preferable.[19] In the case of competent beings' making the judgement that their never existing would have been preferable, he allows that it be merely *consistent* with reason (that is, *not irrational*). Although it is much easier for a judgement to satisfy the requirement that it be consistent with reason, it is a fact of human psychology that very rarely do people—even those enduring considerable hardships—prefer not to have existed. The result is that on Professor Feinberg's view, most beings who are brought into existence with disabilities which although not so bad as to make life worth ending are nonetheless severe cannot be said to be harmed. One can only be harmed if it would have been preferable that one did not come into existence, and on his interpretation of this requirement it is met only very rarely.

The reason why this account conflicts with my distinction between present-life cases and future-life cases is that implicit in it is the requirement that we make judgements about future-life cases through the lens of present-life cases. Either life has to be so bad that it would *not be worth continuing*—Professor Feinberg's standard for proxy decisions—or it has to be the case that *already existing people* with that disability would prefer never to have come into existence—his standard for those whose disabilities do not impair their competence to decide (retrospectively!) for themselves.

---

[19] 'Wrongful Life and the Counterfactual Element in Harming', 22.

However, it is precisely because Professor Feinberg's account requires us to adopt the perspective of already existing people that it is inadequate. In asking whether a life is worth starting, we should not have to consider whether it would not be worth continuing. Nor should we have to appeal to the preferences of already existing people about their own lives to make judgements about future lives. As I shall show in the second section of the next chapter, self-assessments of one's life's quality are unreliable.

Although I reject Professor Feinberg's account of when it is preferable not to come into existence, I agree that we can understand the notion of harming somebody by bringing him into existence, in terms of the preferability of either existing or never existing. That is to say, one harms somebody by bringing him into existence if his existence is such that never existing would have been preferable. Similarly, a person is not harmed by being brought into existence if his existence is such that it is preferable to never existing. The question to which we must now turn, then, is 'When is never existing preferable?' Put another way, 'When does coming into existence harm?' Alternatively we can ask, 'When is coming into existence bad while never coming into existence not bad?' The answer, I shall now argue, is 'Always'.

WHY COMING INTO EXISTENCE IS ALWAYS A HARM

There is a common assumption in the literature about future possible people that, all things being equal, one does no wrong by bringing into existence people whose lives will be good on balance. This assumption rests on another—namely that being brought into existence (with decent life prospects) is a benefit (even though not being brought into existence is not a harm). I shall argue that the underlying assumption is erroneous. Being brought into existence is not a benefit but always a harm. When I say that coming into existence is *always* a harm, I do not mean that it is necessarily a harm. As will become apparent, my argument does not apply to those hypothetical cases in which a life contains only good and no bad. About such an existence I say that it is neither a harm nor a benefit and we should be indifferent between such an existence and never existing. But no lives are like this. All lives contain some bad. Coming into existence with such a life is always a harm. Many people will find this deeply unsettling claim to be counter-intuitive and will wish to dismiss it. For this reason, I propose not only to defend the claim, but also to suggest why people might be resistant to it.

As a matter of fact, bad things happen to all of us. No life is without hardship. It is easy to think of the millions who live a life of poverty or of those who live much of their lives with some disability. Some of us are lucky enough to be spared these fates, but most of us who are, nonetheless suffer ill-health at some stage during our lives. Often the suffering is excruciating, even if it is in our final days. Some are condemned by nature to years of frailty. We *all* face death.[20] We infrequently contemplate the harms that await any new-born child—pain, disappointment, anxiety, grief, and death. For any given child we cannot predict what form these harms will take or how severe they will be, but we can be sure that at least some of them will occur.[21] None of this befalls the non-existent. Only existers suffer harm.

Optimists will be quick to note that I have not told the whole story. Not only bad things but also good things happen only to those who exist. Pleasure, joy, and satisfaction can only be had by existers. Thus, the cheerful will say, we must weigh up the pleasures of life against the evils. As long as the former outweigh

[20] Here I assume the ordinary view that death is a harm. There is a rich philosophical literature on the ancient challenge to this view, which I shall consider (too briefly) in Chapter 7. Those who think that death does not harm the person who dies may simply leave death off my list of harms.
[21] Only those who die very soon after coming into existence are spared much of these harms, but obviously are not spared death.

the latter, the life is worth living. Coming into being with such a life is, on this view, a benefit.

The asymmetry of pleasure and pain

However, this conclusion does not follow. This is because there is a crucial difference between harms (such as pains) and benefits (such as pleasures) which entails that existence has no advantage over, but does have disadvantages relative to, non-existence.[22] Consider pains and pleasures as exemplars of harms and benefits. It is uncontroversial to say that

(1) the presence of pain is bad,
and that
(2) the presence of pleasure is good.

However, such a symmetrical evaluation does not seem to apply to the *absence* of pain and pleasure, for it strikes me as true that

(3) the absence of pain is good, even if that good is not enjoyed by anyone,
whereas
(4) the absence of pleasure is not bad unless there is somebody for whom this absence is a deprivation.

Now it might be asked how the absence of pain could be good if that good is not enjoyed by anybody. Absent pain, it might be said, cannot be good *for* anybody, if nobody exists for whom it can be good. This, however, is to dismiss (3) too quickly.

The judgement made in (3) is made *with reference to the (potential) interests of a person* who either does or does not exist. To this it

---

[22] The term 'non-existence' is multiply ambiguous. It can be applied to those who never exist and to those who do not currently exist. The latter can be divided further into those who do not yet exist and those who are no longer existing. In the current context I am using 'non-existence' to denote those who never exist. Joel Feinberg has argued that the not yet existent and the no longer existent can be harmed. I embrace that view. What I have to say here applies only to the never existent.

might be objected that because (3) is part of the scenario under which this person never exists, (3) cannot say anything about an existing person. This objection would be mistaken because (3) can say something about a counterfactual case in which a person who does actually exist never did exist. Of the pain of an existing person, (3) says that the absence of this pain would have been good even if this could only have been achieved by the absence of the person who now suffers it. In other words, judged in terms of the interests of a person who now exists, the absence of the pain would have been good even though this person would then not have existed. Consider next what (3) says of the absent pain of one who never exists—of pain, the absence of which is ensured by not making a potential person actual. Claim (3) says that this absence is good when judged in terms of the interests of the person who would otherwise have existed. We may not know who that person would have been, but we can still say that whoever that person would have been, the avoidance of his or her pains is good when judged in terms of his or her potential interests. If there is any (obviously loose) sense in which the absent pain is good *for* the person who could have existed but does not exist, this is it. Clearly (3) does not entail the absurd literal claim that there is some actual person for whom the absent pain is good.[23]

In support of the asymmetry between (3) and (4), it can be shown that it has considerable explanatory power. It explains at least four other asymmetries that are quite plausible. Sceptics, when they see where this leads, may begin to question the plausibility of these other asymmetries and may want to know what support (beyond the asymmetry above) can be provided for them. Were I to provide such support, the sceptics would

---

[23] One *could* (logically) make symmetrical claims about the absence of pleasure—that, when judged in terms of the (potential) interests of a person who does or does not exist, this absence of pleasure is bad. However, (4) suggests that this symmetrical claim, although logically possible, is actually false. I shall defend (4) later. For now my aim has been only to show that (3) is not incoherent.

then ask for a defence of these further supporting considerations. Every argument must have some justificatory end. I cannot hope to convince those who take the rejection of my conclusion as axiomatic. All I can show is that those who accept some quite plausible views are led to my conclusion. These plausible views include four other asymmetries, which I shall now outline.

First, the asymmetry between (3) and (4) is the best explanation for the view that while there is a duty to avoid bringing suffering people into existence, there is no duty to bring happy people into being. In other words, the reason why we think that there is a duty not to bring suffering people into existence is that the presence of this suffering would be bad (for the sufferers) and the absence of the suffering is good (even though there is nobody to enjoy the absence of suffering). In contrast to this, we think that there is no duty to bring happy people into existence because while their pleasure would be good for them, its absence would not be bad for them (given that there would be nobody who would be deprived of it).

It might be objected that there is an alternative explanation for the view about our procreational duties—one that does not appeal to my claim about the asymmetry between (3) and (4). It might be suggested that the reason why we have a duty to avoid bringing suffering people into being, but not a duty to bring happy people into existence, is that we have negative duties to avoid harm but no corresponding positive duties to bring about happiness. Judgements about our procreational duties are thus like judgements about all other duties. Now I agree that for those who deny that we have any positive duties, this would indeed be an alternative explanation to the one I have provided. However, even of those who do think that we have positive duties only a few also think that amongst these is a duty to bring happy people into existence.

It might now be suggested that there is also an alternative explanation why those who *do* accept positive duties do not usually think that these include a duty to bring happy people into existence. It is usually thought that our positive duties cannot include a duty to create lots of pleasure if that would require significant sacrifice on our part. Given that having children involves considerable sacrifice (at least to the pregnant woman), this, and not asymmetry, is the best explanation for why there is no duty to bring happy people into existence.

The problem, though, with this alternative explanation is that it implies that in the absence of this sacrifice[24] we *would* have a duty to bring happy people into existence. In other words, it would be wrong not to create such people if we could create them without great cost to ourselves. But this presupposes that the duty under discussion is an all-things-considered duty. However, the interests of potential people cannot ground even a defeasible duty to bring them into existence. Put another way, the asymmetry of procreative (all-things-considered) duties rests on another asymmetry—an asymmetry of procreative moral *reasons*. According to this asymmetry, although we have a strong moral reason, grounded in the interests of potential people,[25] to avoid creating unhappy people, we have no strong moral reason (grounded in the interests of potential people) to create happy people.[26] It follows that although the extent of the sacrifice may be relevant to other positive duties,

[24] Or even in its presence, if it is not thought to be great enough to defeat this duty. Just how great must a sacrifice be to prevent a positive duty arising is a complex and hotly disputed matter that I shall not consider here. There are not a few people who think that the extent of the sacrifice that can be required of us is quite considerable. See, for example, Singer, Peter, *Practical Ethics* 2nd edn. (Cambridge: Cambridge University Press, 1993). Notice, by the way, that although Peter Singer's conclusions about the extent of our positive duties are radically counterintuitive, that counterintuitiveness is not usually thought to suffice as an argument against his position. Curiously, though, there is much less hesitance to treat my conclusions as a *reductio* of my argument. I shall say more about this in Chapter 7.

[25] The condition that the moral reason (or duty) be grounded in the interests of the potential person is an important one. Those who find plausibility in the claim that we have a reason to create happy people tend to be motivated by impersonal considerations—such as there being more happiness in the world. But these are not considerations about the interests of the potential person.

[26] Jeff McMahan says that 'the view that there is no strong moral reason to cause a person to exist just because his life would contain much good. . .is deeply intuitive and probably impossible to dislodge.' *The Ethics of Killing: Problems at the Margins of Life* (New York: Oxford University Press, 2002) 300.

this is moot in the case of a purported duty to bring happy people into existence.

There is a second support for my claim about the asymmetry between (3) and (4). Whereas it is strange (if not incoherent) to give as a reason for having a child that the child one has will thereby be benefited,[27] it is not strange to cite a potential child's interests as a basis for avoiding bringing a child into existence. If having children were done for the purpose of thereby benefiting those children, then there would be greater moral reason for at least many people to have more children. In contrast to this, our concern for the welfare of potential children who would suffer is a sound basis for deciding *not* to have the child. If absent pleasures were bad irrespective of whether they were bad for anybody, then having children for their own sakes would not be odd. And if it were not the case that absent pains are good even where they are not good for anybody, then we could not say that it would be good to avoid bringing suffering children into existence.

Thirdly, support for the asymmetry between (3) and (4) can be drawn from a related asymmetry, this time in our retrospective judgements. Bringing people into existence as well as failing to bring people into existence can be regretted. However, only bringing people into existence can be regretted *for* the sake of the person whose existence was contingent on our decision. This is *not* because those who are not brought into existence are indeterminate. Instead it is because they never exist. We can regret, for the sake of an indeterminate but existent person that a benefit was not bestowed on him or her, but we cannot regret, for the sake of somebody who never exists and thus cannot thereby be deprived, a good that this never existent person never experiences. One might grieve about not having had children, but not because the children that one could have had have been deprived of existence. Remorse about not having children is remorse for

---

[27] In other words, it is odd to suggest that one can have a child for that child's sake.

ourselves—sorrow about having missed childbearing and child-rearing experiences. However, we do regret having brought into existence a child with an unhappy life, and we regret it for the child's sake, even if also for our own sakes. The reason why we do not lament our failure to bring somebody into existence is because absent pleasures are not bad.

Finally, support for the asymmetry between (3) and (4) can be found in the asymmetrical judgements about (a) (distant) suffering and (b) uninhabited portions of the earth or the universe. Whereas, at least when we think of them, we rightly are sad for inhabitants of a foreign land whose lives are characterized by suffering, when we hear that some island is unpopulated, we are not similarly sad for the happy people who, had they existed, would have populated this island. Similarly, nobody really mourns for those who do not exist on Mars, feeling sorry for potential such beings that they cannot enjoy life.[28] Yet, if we knew that there were sentient life on Mars but that Martians were suffering, we would regret this for them. The claim here need not (but could) be the strong one that we would regret their very existence. The fact that we would regret the suffering *within* their life is sufficient to support the asymmetry I am defending. The point is that we regret suffering but not the absent pleasures of those who could have existed.

Now it might be objected that just as we do not regret the absent pleasures of those who could have existed, we do not take joy in the absent pain of those who could have existed. For if we did, the objection goes, we should be overjoyed by the amount of pain that is avoided, given how few of all the possible people

[28] That most people do not even think about the absent lives on Mars is itself revealing. Once forced to think about these issues some will claim that they regret absent Martian pleasure. Whether or not they do, I cannot see how one could regret it for the sake of the (non-existent) Martians who would otherwise enjoy that pleasure. It is curious, however, how some people will begin to say that they do feel sorry for the absent Martians once they realize that not doing so supports asymmetry and thus the conclusion that coming into existence is always a harm. However, saying this and its making sense are two different matters.

ever become actual, and thus how much pain is avoided. But joy is not the appropriate contrast to regret. Although we regret the suffering of distant others, at least when we think about them, we are not usually overcome with melancholy about it.[29] Thus the important question is not whether we feel joy—the opposite of melancholy—about absent pains but whether the absent pain is the opposite of regrettable—what we might call 'welcome' or simply 'good'. The answer, I have suggested, is affirmative. If we are asked whether the absent suffering is a good feature of never existing, we would have to say that it is.

I have shown that the asymmetry between (3) and (4) explains four other asymmetries. Given that these other asymmetries are widely endorsed, we have good grounds for thinking that the asymmetry between (3) and (4) is also widely accepted. That it is so is not evidence of its truth, for the multitude can be and often are wrong. However, it does show that my starting point should have broad appeal.

The judgements supported by the asymmetry of (3) and (4) are not universally shared. For example, positive utilitarians—who are interested not only in minimizing pain but also in maximizing pleasure—would tend to lament the absence of additional possible pleasure even if there were nobody deprived of that pleasure. On their view, there *is* a duty to bring people into existence if that would increase happiness. This is not to say that all positive utilitarians *must* reject the view about the asymmetry of (3) and (4). Positive utilitarians who are sympathetic to the asymmetry could draw a distinction between (i) promoting the happiness of people (that exist, or will exist independently of one's choices) and (ii) increasing happiness by making people. This is the now famous distinction between (i) making people happy and (ii) making happy people. Positive utilitarians who draw this distinction could then,

---

[29] That we do not have the more marked reaction is probably the result of a psychological defence mechanism.

consistent with positive utilitarianism, judge only (i) to be a requirement of morality. This is the preferable version of positive utilitarianism. Taking (ii) also to be a requirement of morality mistakenly assumes that the value of happiness is primary and the value of persons is derivative from this. However, it is not the case that people are valuable because they add extra happiness. Instead extra happiness is valuable because it is good for people—because it makes people's lives go better. To think otherwise is to think that people are mere means to the production of happiness. Or, to use another famous image, it is to treat persons as mere vessels of happiness. But unlike a mere vessel, which is indifferent to how much of a valued substance it contains, a person cares about how much happiness he has.

If my arguments so far are sound, then the view about the asymmetry between harm and benefit is both compelling and widespread. My argument will proceed by showing how, given the asymmetry between harm and benefit, it follows that coming into existence is always a harm. In the concluding chapter (Chapter 7) I shall consider the objection of those who, when they see where the asymmetry leads, would rather give it up than accept the conclusion that coming into existence is always a harm. The objection is that the conclusions of my argument are more counter-intuitive than giving up the asymmetry would be, and thus if either of these has to be sacrificed it should be the asymmetry. I delay discussing this objection until the final chapter because it applies not only to the counter-intuitiveness of my conclusion so far but also to other counter-intuitive conclusions for which I shall argue in coming chapters. (Those who are impatient to see this objection addressed may turn to the opening section—'Countering the counter-intuitiveness objection'—of Chapter 7.)

To show why, given the asymmetry I have defended, it is always a harm to come into existence it is necessary to compare two scenarios, one (A) in which X exists and one (B) in which X never exists. This, along with the views already mentioned, is represented diagrammatically in Figure 2.1.

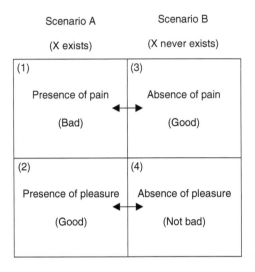

Figure 2.1.

If I am correct then it is uncontroversially the case that (1) is bad and (2) is good. However, in accordance with the considerations mentioned above, (3) is good even though there is nobody to enjoy the good, but (4) is not bad because there is nobody who is deprived of the absent benefits.

Drawing on my earlier defence of the asymmetry, we should note that alternative ways of evaluating (3) and (4), according to which a symmetry between pain and pleasure is preserved, must fail, at least if common important judgements are to be preserved. The first option is shown in Figure 2.2.

Here, to preserve symmetry, the absence of pleasure (4) has been termed 'bad'. This judgement is too strong because if the absence of pleasure in Scenario B is 'bad' rather than 'not bad' then

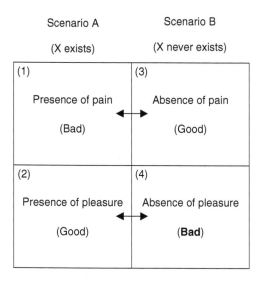

	Scenario A (X exists)	Scenario B (X never exists)
	(1) Presence of pain (Bad)	(3) Absence of pain (Good)
	(2) Presence of pleasure (Good)	(4) Absence of pleasure (**Bad**)

Figure 2.2.

we should have to regret, for X's sake, that X did not come into existence. But it is not regrettable.

The second way to effect a symmetrical evaluation of pleasure and pain is shown in Figure 2.3.

To preserve symmetry in this case, the absence of pain (3) has been termed 'not bad' rather than 'good', and the absence of pleasure (4) has been termed 'not good' rather than 'not bad'. On one interpretation, 'not bad' is equivalent to 'good', and 'not good' is equivalent to 'bad'. But this is not the interpretation that is operative in this matrix, for if it were, it would not differ from, and would have the same shortcomings as, the previous matrix. 'Not bad', in Figure 2.3, therefore must mean 'not bad, but not good either'. Interpreted in this way, however, it is too weak. Avoiding the pains of existence is more than merely 'not bad'. It is good.

Judging the absence of pleasure to be 'not good' is also too weak in that it does not say enough. Of course the absence of pleasure is

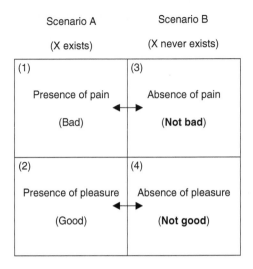

Figure 2.3.

not what we would call good. However, the important question, when the absence of pleasure involves no deprivation for anybody, is whether it is also 'not bad' or whether it is 'bad'. The answer, I suggest, is that it is 'not good, but not bad either' rather than 'not good, but bad'. Because 'not bad' is a more informative evaluation than 'not good', that is the one I prefer. However, even those who wish to stick with 'not good' will not thereby succeed in restoring symmetry. If pain is bad and pleasure is good, but the absence of pain is good and the absence of pleasure not good, then there is no symmetry between pleasure and pain.

Comparing existing with never existing

Having rejected alternative evaluations, I return to my original diagram. To determine the relative advantages and disadvantages of coming into existence and never coming to be, we need to compare (1) with (3), and (2) with (4). In the first comparison we see that non-existence is preferable to existence. Non-existence has an advantage over existence. In the second comparison, however, the pleasures of the existent, although good, are not an advantage over non-existence, because the absence of pleasures is not bad. For the good to be an advantage over non-existence, it would have to have been the case that its absence were bad.

To this it might be objected that 'good' *is* an advantage over 'not bad' because a pleasurable sensation is better than a neutral state. The mistake underlying this objection, however, is that it treats the absence of pleasure in Scenario B as though it were akin to the absence of pleasure in Scenario A—a possibility not reflected in my matrix, but which is implicit in (4) of my original description of asymmetry. There I said that the absence of pleasure is not bad *unless there is somebody for whom this absence is a deprivation.* The implication here is that where an absent pleasure is a deprivation it is bad. Now, obviously, when I say that it is bad, I do not mean that it is bad in the same way that the presence of pain is bad.[30] What is meant is that the absent pleasure is relatively (rather than intrinsically) bad. In other words, it is *worse* than the presence of pleasure. But that is because X exists in Scenario A. It would have been better had X had the pleasure of which he is deprived. Instead of a pleasurable mental state, X has a neutral state. Absent pleasures in Scenario B, by contrast, are not neutral states of some person. They are no states of a person at all. Although the pleasures in A are better than the absent pleasures in A, the pleasures in A are not better than the absent pleasures in B.

The point may be made another way. Just as I am not talking about intrinsic badness when I say that absent pleasures that deprive are bad, so I am not speaking about intrinsic 'not badness'—neutrality—when I speak about absent pleasures that do not deprive. Just as absent pleasures that do deprive are 'bad' in

---

[30] The only time it would be bad in that sense is where the absence of pleasure is actually painful.

the sense of 'worse', so absent pleasures that do not deprive are 'not bad' in the sense of 'not worse'. They are not worse than the presence of pleasures. It follows that the presence of pleasures is not better, and therefore that the presence of pleasures is not an advantage over absent pleasures that do not deprive.

Some people have difficulty understanding how (2) is not an advantage over (4). They should consider an analogy which, because it involves the comparison of two existent people is unlike the comparison between existence and non-existence in *this* way, but which nonetheless may be instructive. S (Sick) is prone to regular bouts of illness. Fortunately for him, he is also so constituted that he recovers quickly. H (Healthy) lacks the capacity for quick recovery, but he *never* gets sick. It is bad for S that he gets sick and it is good for him that he recovers quickly. It is good that H never gets sick, but it is not bad that he lacks the capacity to heal speedily. The capacity for quick recovery, although a good for S, is not a real advantage over H. This is because the absence of that capacity is not bad for H. This, in turn, is because the absence of that capacity is not a deprivation for H. H is not worse off than he would have been had he had the recuperative powers of S. S is not better off than H in any way, even though S is better off than he himself would have been had he lacked the capacity for rapid recovery.

It might be objected that the analogy is tendentious. It is obvious that it is better to be Healthy than to be Sick. The objection is that if I treat these as analogies for never existing and existing respectively, then I bias the discussion toward my favoured conclusion. But the problem with this objection, if it is taken alone, is that it could be levelled at all analogies. The point of an analogy is to find a case (such as H and S) where matters are clear and thereby to shed some light on a disputed case (such as Scenarios A and B in Fig. 2.1). Tendentiousness, then, is not the core issue. Instead, the real question is whether or not the analogy is a good one.

One reason why it might be thought not to be a good analogy is that whereas pleasure (in Fig. 2.1) is an *intrinsic* good, the capacity for quick recovery is but an *instrumental* good. It might be argued further that it would be impossible to provide an analogy involving two existing people (such as H and S) that could show one of the people not to be disadvantaged by lacking some *intrinsic* good that the other has. Since the only unambiguous cases of an actual person lacking a good and not thereby being disadvantaged are cases involving *instrumental* goods, the difference between intrinsic and instrumental goods might be thought to be relevant.

This, however, is unconvincing, because there is a deeper explanation of why absent intrinsic goods could always be thought to be bad in analogies involving only existing people. Given that these people exist, the absence of any intrinsic good could always be thought to constitute a deprivation for them. In analogies that compare two existing people the only way to simulate the absence of deprivation is by considering instrumental goods.[31] Because (3) and (4) make it explicit that the presence or absence of deprivation is crucial, it seems entirely fair that the analogy should test this feature and can ignore the differences between intrinsic and instrumental goods.

Notice, in any event, that the analogy need not be read as proving that quadrant (2) is good and that quadrant (4) is not bad. That asymmetry was established in the previous section. Instead, the analogy could be interpreted as showing how, given the asymmetry, (2) is not an advantage over (4), whereas (1) is a disadvantage relative to (3). It would thereby show that Scenario B is preferable to Scenario A.

We can ascertain the relative advantages and disadvantages of existence and non-existence in another way, still in my original matrix, but by comparing (2) with (3) and (4) with (1). There are

---

[31] Any instructive analogy for Scenarios A and B would have to involve a comparison of two existing people. An analogy involving an existing and non-existing person would be no clearer than the case we are trying to illuminate. Thus we cannot be required to consider analogies that compare a person's existence with his never existing.

benefits both to existing and non-existing. It is good that existers enjoy their pleasures. It is also good that pains are avoided through non-existence. However, that is only part of the picture. Because there is nothing bad about never coming into existence, but there is something bad about coming into existence, it seems that all things considered non-existence is preferable.

One of the realizations which emerges from some of the reflections so far is that the cost-benefit analysis of the cheerful—whereby one weighs up (1) the pleasures of life against (2) the evils—is unconvincing as a comparison between the desirability of existence and never existing. The analysis of the cheerful is mistaken for a number of reasons:

First, it makes the wrong comparison. If we want to determine whether non-existence is preferable to existence, or vice versa, then we must compare the left- and the right-hand sides of the diagram, which represent the alternative scenarios in which X exists and in which X never exists. Comparing the upper and the lower quadrants on the left does not tell us whether Scenario A is better than Scenario B or vice versa. That is unless quadrants (3) and (4) are rendered irrelevant. One way in which that would be so is if they were both valued as 'zero'. On this assumption A can be thought to be better than B if (2) is greater than (1), or to put it another way, if (2) minus (1) is greater than zero. But this poses a second problem. To value quadrants (3) and (4) at zero is to attach no positive value to (3) and this is incompatible with the asymmetry for which I have argued. (It would be to adopt the symmetry of Fig. 2.3.)

Another problem with calculating whether A or B is better by looking only at (1) and (2), subtracting the former from the latter, is that it seems to ignore the difference, mentioned earlier, between a 'life worth starting' and a 'life worth continuing'. The cheerful tell us that existence is better than non-existence if (2) is greater than (1). But what is meant by 'non-existence' here? Does it mean 'never existing' or 'ceasing to exist'? Those who look only at (1) and

(2) do not seem to be distinguishing between never existing and ceasing to exist. For them, a life is worth living (that is, both starting and continuing) if (2) is greater than (1), otherwise it is not worth living (that is, neither worth starting nor continuing). The problem with this, I have already argued, is that there is good reason to distinguish between them. For a life to be not worth continuing, it must be worse than it need be for it not to be worth starting.[32] Those who consider not only Scenario A but also Scenario B clearly are considering which lives are worth starting. To determine which lives are worth continuing, Scenario A would have to be compared with a third scenario, in which X ceases to exist.[33]

Finally, the quality of a life is not determined simply by subtracting the bad from the good. As I shall show in the first section of the next chapter, assessing the quality of a life is much more complicated than this.

Now some people might accept the asymmetry represented in Figure 2.1, agree that we need to compare Scenario A with Scenario B, but deny that this leads to the conclusion that B is always preferable to A—that is, deny that coming into existence is always a harm. The argument is that we must assign positive or negative (or neutral) values to each of the quadrants, and that if we assign them in what those advancing this view take to be the most reasonable way, we find that coming into existence is sometimes preferable (see Fig. 2.4).[34]

---

[32] Those who consider only Scenario A *could* offer different judgements about when life is 'worth starting' and when it is 'worth continuing'. They could do so by setting different thresholds. Thus, they might say that for a life to be worth continuing, (2) need only just outweigh (1), but for a life to be worth starting, (2) must be significantly greater than (1). Although those who consider only Scenario A could do this, there is no evidence that they are doing it. They seem to treat the judgements alike. In any event, even if they could rectify this, their position would still succumb to the other objections I am raising.

[33] In this scenario, which we might call Scenario C, the absence of pain would be 'good' and the absence of pleasure would be 'bad'.

[34] I am grateful to Robert Segall for raising this challenge.

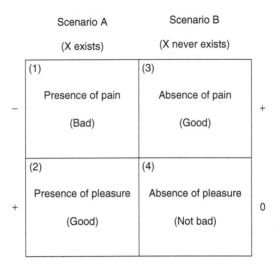

	Scenario A (X exists)	Scenario B (X never exists)	
−	**(1)** Presence of pain (Bad)	**(3)** Absence of pain (Good)	+
+	**(2)** Presence of pleasure (Good)	**(4)** Absence of pleasure (Not bad)	0

Figure 2.4.

Quadrant (1) must be negative, because it is bad, and quadrants (2) and (3) must be positive because they are good. (I assume that (3) must be *as* good as (1) is bad. That is, if (1) = −n, then (3) = +n). Since (4) is not bad (and not good either), it should be neither positive nor negative but rather neutral.

Employing the value assignments of Figure 2.4 we add (1) and (2) in order to determine the value of A, and then compare this with the sum of (3) and (4), which is the value of B. Doing this, we find that A is preferable to B where (2) is more than twice the value of (1).[35] There are numerous problems with this. For instance, as I shall show in the first section of the next chapter, it is not only the ratio of pleasure to pain that determines the quality of a life, but also the sheer quantity of pain. Once a certain threshold of pain is passed, no amount of pleasure can compensate for it.

[35] Where (2) is only twice the value of (1), A and B have equal value and thus neither coming into existence nor never coming into existence is preferable.

But the best way to show that Figure 2.4 is mistaken is to apply the reasoning behind Figure 2.4 to the analogy of H (Healthy) and S (Sick) mentioned earlier.

	S	H	
−	(1) Presence of sickness (Bad)	(3) Absence of sickness (Good)	+
+	(2) Presence of capacity for quick recovery (Good)	(4) Absence of capacity for quick recovery (Not bad)	0

Figure 2.5.

Following Figure 2.5, it would be better to be S than H if the value of (2) were more than twice the value of (1). (This presumably would be the case where the amount of suffering that (2) saves S is more than twice the amount S actually suffers.) But this cannot be right, for surely it is *always* better to be H (a person who never gets sick and is thus not disadvantaged by lacking the capacity for quick recovery). The whole point is that (2) is *good for* S but does not constitute an advantage over H. By assigning a positive charge to (2) and a '0' to (4), Figure 2.5 suggests that (2) is an advantage over (4), but it quite clearly is not. The assignment of values in Figure 2.5, and hence also in Figure 2.4, must be mistaken.[36]

---

[36] To take the implications of the value assignments in Fig. 2.5 for Fig. 2.4 as evidence that the analogy between the two cases must be inapt is another instance of treating the avoidance of my conclusion as axiomatic.

Now it might be asked what the *correct* value assignments are, but I want to resist that question because it is the wrong one to ask. Figure 2.1 is intended to show why it is always preferable not to come into existence. It shows that coming into existence has disadvantages relative to never coming into existence whereas the positive features of existing are not advantages over never existing. Scenario B is always better than Scenario A for much the same reason that it is always preferable to be H rather than S. Figure 2.1 is not meant to be a guide to determining *how* bad it is to come into existence.

There is a difference, I have indicated, between (a) saying that coming into existence is always a harm and (b) saying how great a harm it is. So far I have argued only for the first claim. The magnitude of the harm of existence varies from person to person, and in the next chapter I shall argue that the harm is very substantial for everybody. However, it must be stressed that one can endorse the view that coming into existence is always a harm and yet deny that the harm is great. Similarly, if one thinks that the harm of existence is not great, one cannot infer from that that existence is preferable to non-existence.

This recognition is important for warding off another potential objection to my argument. One of the implications of my argument is that a life filled with good and containing only the most minute quantity of bad—a life of utter bliss adulterated only by the pain of a single pin-prick—is worse than no life at all. The objection is that this is implausible. Understanding the distinction between (a) coming into existence being a harm and (b) how great a harm it is, enables one to see why this implication is not so implausible. It is true of the person enjoying this charmed life marred only by a single brief sharp pain, that as pleasant as his life is, it has no advantages over never existing. Yet coming into existence has the disadvantage of the single pain. We can acknowledge that the harm of coming into existence is minuscule without denying that it is harm. Setting aside the matter of whether coming into existence is a harm, who would deny that a brief sharp pain is a harm, even if only a minor one? And if one acknowledges that it is a harm—one that would have been avoided had that life not begun—why should one deny that a life begun at that cost is a harm, even if only a minor one? Think again of the analogy of S and H. If S gets sick only once, and then only has a headache that quickly subsides, it is still better to be H (even though not that much better). If all lives were as free of suffering as that of the imagined person who suffers only a pin-prick, the harms of coming into existence would easily be outweighed by the benefits to others (including the potential parents) of that person coming into existence. In the real world, however, there are no lives even nearly this charmed.[37]

Other asymmetries

I have argued that pleasure and pain are asymmetrical in a way that makes coming into existence always a harm. After arguing in the coming chapter that this harm is substantial, I shall discuss, in Chapter 4, the implications of all this for procreation. It should be clear now, however, that the idea that coming into existence is always a serious harm raises a problem for procreation. Procreation can be challenged in many other ways too, but the arguments of Christoph Fehige[38] and Seana Shiffrin[39] have interesting parallels with my argument.

Consider Seana Shiffrin's argument first. The understanding of benefit and harm implicit in my argument is similar to that which she makes explicit in hers. She understands benefit and harm non-comparatively. That is to say, she understands them not as two

[37] I discuss the implications of this in Chapter 4 ('Having Children').
[38] Fehige, Christoph, 'A Pareto Principle for Possible People', in Fehige, Christoph, and Wessels, Ulla, eds., *Preferences* (Berlin: Walter de Gruyter, 1998) 508–43.
[39] Shiffrin, Seana Valentine, 'Wrongful Life, Procreative Responsibility, and the Significance of Harm', *Legal Theory*, 5 (1999) 117–48.

ends of a scale or as shifts up and down such a scale. Instead she understands them as absolute conditions of, respectively, a positive and a negative kind. Moreover, her argument, like mine, appeals to an asymmetry between benefits and harms, albeit a different asymmetry. She says that in the absence of evidence of a person's wishes to the contrary, it is permissible, perhaps obligatory, to inflict a lesser harm on that person in order to prevent a greater harm. By contrast, it would be wrong to inflict a harm that would yield a greater (pure) benefit.[40] Thus, we take it to be acceptable to break an unconscious (non-consenting) person's arm in order to prevent a greater harm, such as death, to that person. (This is the 'rescue case'.) However, we would condemn breaking that person's arm in order to secure some greater benefit, such as 'supernormal memory, a useful store of encyclopedic knowledge, twenty IQ points worth of extra intellectual ability, or the ability to consume immoderate amounts of alcohol or fat without side effects'.[41] (Call this the 'pure benefit case'.)

Since all existers suffer harm, procreation always causes harm. Professor Shiffrin is prepared to grant (for the sake of argument?) that 'being created *can* benefit a person.'[42] However, in accordance with the asymmetry just mentioned, we may not inflict the harm in order to secure the benefit. Although existing people can sometimes authorize our inflicting harm in order to secure some benefit for them, we can never obtain the consent of those whom we bring into existence before we create them. Nor can we presume hypothetical consent, she argues. There are four reasons for this.[43] First, the person is not harmed if we fail to create him or her. Secondly, the harms of existence may be severe. Thirdly, the harms of life cannot be escaped without considerable cost. Finally,

---

[40] By 'pure benefit' she means 'benefits that are only goods and which are not also removals from or preventions of harm' (ibid.124). The intrinsic pleasures to which I refer in Chapter 3 would be instances of 'pure benefit' whereas the relief pleasures to which I refer are instances of 'removals from harm'.

[41] Ibid. 127.   [42] Ibid. 119.   [43] Ibid. 131–3.

the hypothetical consent is not based on the individual's values or attitudes towards risk.

There are some interesting differences between Professor Shiffrin's argument and mine. Her argument, at least on the surface, does not preclude treating life's goods as advantages over non-existence (although, as I shall show, it does not require treating them as such). On her view, even if pleasures and other goods enjoyed by existers are advantages over non-existence, they are not advantages that we may secure at the costs of existence.[44]

Nor does her basic argument presuppose the asymmetry I have defended. We can see this by comparing two scenarios that involve existing people and that are not characterized by the asymmetry in Figure 2.1. The first of these scenarios is one in which a pure benefit is bestowed at the cost of a harm and the other is one in which that harm is avoided at the cost of the pure benefit. Following the pattern of the earlier matrices, we might represent this as shown in Figure 2.6.

My asymmetry does not apply in such a case, yet on Professor Shiffrin's asymmetry we would not be warranted in inflicting (1) to secure (2). Put another way, we may not bring about Scenario A over Scenario B (absent the person's consent). Even when applied to cases of procreation, where (I have argued) my asymmetry does apply, Professor Shiffrin's prioritizing of B over A is not based on my asymmetry but rather on hers.

This does not mean that my asymmetry is unconnected with her argument, and it certainly does not mean that my asymmetry is incompatible with it. We find, first, that at least one feature of my asymmetry makes her case against procreation even stronger

---

[44] Or at least not without being prepared to compensate for the harms. Seana Shiffrin is a little reticent about ruling out procreation entirely, although her argument does seem to entail this conclusion and one suspects that she would embrace it. She explicitly defends only the weaker claim that procreation is not a 'straightforward, morally innocent endeavor' (ibid. 118).

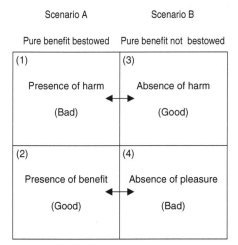

	Scenario A	Scenario B
	Pure benefit bestowed	Pure benefit not bestowed
	(1) Presence of harm (Bad)	(3) Absence of harm (Good)
	(2) Presence of benefit (Good)	(4) Absence of pleasure (Bad)

Figure 2.6.

than her case against other bestowals of pure benefit that cause harm. Professor Shiffrin notes that procreation is not like cases of inflicting a harm in order to rescue somebody because 'if the benefit bestowed by creation is not conferred, the nonexistent person will not experience its absence.' She might have added that in this regard procreation is unlike not only the rescue case, but also non-procreative cases of bestowing pure benefit at the cost of harm. Implicitly recognized here is that the absent benefit when somebody is not brought into existence is not bad (quadrant 4 of Fig. 2.1). It is less clear how Professor Shiffrin views the claim in quadrant (3) in Figure 2.1—that the absence of harm when somebody is not created is good. However, I suggest that that claim too would strengthen her case against procreation (although I recognize that she may not be aiming to strengthen this case). Procreation would be more threatened if the absent harms were good and not merely neither bad nor good.

In response to Professor Shiffrin's argument, it has been objected that her asymmetry is not needed to explain the pure benefit case—the case where some benefit is bestowed but at the cost of a harm. It has been suggested[45] that in the pure benefit case Seana Shiffrin describes, somebody's rights have been violated (by having his arm broken without his permission), and *this* explains why the benefit may not be bestowed. It can only be bestowed by violating a right not to be harmed. The implicit assumption here is that in the case of procreation nobody's rights are violated, at least so long as the resultant life is one 'worth living'.

One common basis for denying that procreation violates the rights of the person created is that prior to procreation that person does not exist and thus there can be no bearer of the right not to be created. But this may be an unduly narrow view of rights ascription—one that ignores the special features of procreation. If, as I argued in the opening section of this chapter, one *can* be harmed by being brought into existence, one could argue that the right that protects against this kind of harm is a special kind of right—a right that has a bearer only in the breach. Put another way, we might say that one violates a right by performing some action if, as a result of performing this action, there exists some person who is wrongfully harmed. I acknowledge that this is an unusual kind of right, but coming into existence is an unusual case. If one could make sense of such a right, it would then not be an objection to an argument that a person is wrongfully harmed that there was no right not to be.[46]

Those who agree that there is no logical obstacle to a right not to be created might still argue that the pure benefit case fails

<hr>

[45] Wasserman, David, 'Is Every Birth Wrongful? Is Any Birth Morally Required?', DeCamp Bioethics Lecture (Princeton, 2004) unpublished manuscript, 8.

[46] Obviously much more needs to be said about this. I have sketched only the outline of a response. It is not my aim to prove that there is a right not to come into existence, but rather to show that coming into existence is always a harm. Later I shall argue that we have a duty not to cause this harm.

to support the (unqualified) asymmetry that Seana Shiffrin wishes to defend. This is because there are actually two kinds of pure benefit cases (which she does not distinguish). First, there are those involving autonomous beings. They have a right not to be harmed without their consent, even for their benefit. Secondly, there are those involving non-autonomous beings. Although they *could* (logically) also have such a right, it could plausibly be argued that they *do not* (morally) have such a right. Although there are limits on the harms parents may inflict on a child for that child's sake, there certainly are cases where a child's best interests (considering both benefits and harms) may warrant the imposition of a harm. Defenders of procreation might argue that although we may not inflict a harm on an autonomous being without his consent even if this will secure a greater benefit for him, we may sometimes do otherwise in the case of children and, a fortiori, of potential children. It is in response to such a criticism that it becomes helpful for Seana Shiffrin to appeal to my asymmetry or, as she implicitly does, at least to part of it. By denying that somebody's best interests can be served by being brought into existence, she can draw the distinction between children and potential children, and thus ward off the paternalistic objection that parents may inflict the harms of life on a potential child for that child's sake. I have argued that making potential people actual is not in their interests.

Christoph Fehige's argument is arguably even closer to mine than Seana Shiffrin's. He defends and then spells out the implications of a view that he calls 'antifrustrationism' (but which is sometimes called what sounds like its opposite—'frustrationism'). According to this view, a satisfied preference and no preference are equally good. Only an unsatisfied preference is bad. In other words, he argues that although it is good to have fulfilled whatever desires one might have, one is not better off having a fulfilled desire than having no desire at all. By way of example, consider the case in which we 'paint the tree nearest to Sydney Opera house red and give Kate a pill that makes her wish that the tree nearest to Sydney Opera House were red'.[47] Professor Fehige plausibly denies that we do Kate any favour in doing this. She is no better off than had we done nothing. What matters is not that people have satisfied desires but that they do not have unsatisfied ones. It is the avoidance of frustration that is important. There is an asymmetry buried here, as Figure 2.7 shows.

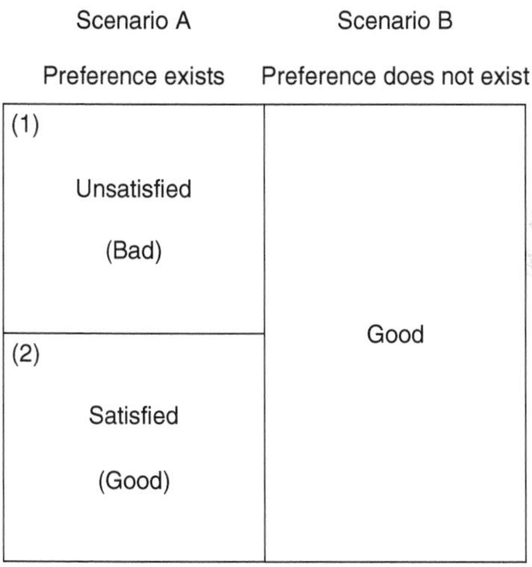

	Scenario A	Scenario B
	Preference exists	Preference does not exist
(1)	Unsatisfied (Bad)	Good
(2)	Satisfied (Good)	

Figure 2.7.

Antifrustrationism implies that it would be better not to create people. Their satisfied preferences will not be better than the absence of their preferences had they not existed. However, their unsatisfied preferences—of which there will be many—are worse than the absence of their preferences if they were not created. (1) is worse than B, but (2) is not better than B.

We can adapt Figure 2.7 to show more clearly its relation to the asymmetry I have defended (see Fig. 2.8).

[47] Fehige, Christoph, 'A Pareto Principle for Possible People', 513–14.

Scenario A	Scenario B
(X exists)	(X never exists)
(1) Preference unsatisfied (Bad)	(3) Absent preference that would have been unsatisfied (in A). (Good)
(2) Preference satisfied (Good)	(4) Absent preference that would have been satisfied (in A). (Good)

Figure 2.8.

In this adaptation, I have taken the liberty of differentiating (3) from (4) even though Professor Fehige does not do so. He treats all absent preferences alike. However, it does not seem that this differentiation is incompatible with his argument. I have also labelled (2), (3), and (4) all as 'good'. This is because Professor Fehige says that absent preferences and satisfied preferences are 'equally good'.[48] If this is the correct reading of Professor Fehige, then his asymmetry is a little different from mine, even though it yields the same result—that Scenario A is worse than Scenario B.

----

[48] Ibid. 508.

However, there may be other ways of reading him. When he says that (2) and Scenario B are 'equally good', he might not mean to describe (3) and (4) as good. He might mean only that (2) is no better than Scenario B. This is exactly what I meant when I described (4) in Figure 2.1 as 'not bad'. I meant that it was no worse than (2). The problem with describing (4) in Figure 2.8 as 'not bad' is that because Professor Fehige seems to treat (3) and (4) as equivalent, (3) would also have to be labelled 'not bad'. If 'not bad' there meant the same as in (4)—that is, 'not worse'—then (3) would not be worse than (1). However, this seems too weak, as I indicated earlier. (3) is better than (1). The alternative, then, is to postulate that if Professor Fehige differentiated (3) and (4) that he would understand them differently. He might understand 'not bad' as meaning something different in the third and fourth quadrants of Figure 2.8. In (3) it would mean 'better' than (1), while in (4) it means 'not worse' than (2). On this reading, we might label (3) as 'good', because 'good' is (sufficiently) better than 'bad'. In this way, Christoph Fehige's asymmetry could be interpreted to be the same as mine.

Whichever of these two readings one adopts, (3) is better than (1), and (4) is not worse than (2). The same is true in Figure 2.1. In both, coming into existence (Scenario A) is worse than never coming into existence (Scenario B).

Against not regretting one's existence

Those who think (with Alfred Lord Tennyson) that it is better to have loved and lost than never to have loved at all[49] might think that they can apply similar reasoning to the case of coming into existence. They might want to say that it is better to have existed and lost (both by suffering within life and then by ceasing to exist) than never to have existed at all. I shall not pass judgement on

[49] Tennyson, Alfred Lord, *In Memoriam*, section 27, stanza 4 (lines 15 and 16).

whether it is indeed better to have loved and lost than never to have loved at all. It suffices to say that even if that claim is true, it does not entail anything about coming into existence. This is because there is a crucial difference between loving and coming into existence. The person who never loves exists without loving and is thus deprived. That, on my account, is 'bad'. (Whether it is *worse* than loving and losing is another question.) By contrast, one who never comes into existence is not deprived of anything. That, I have argued, is 'not bad'.

That coming into existence is a harm is a hard conclusion for most people to swallow. Most people do not regret their very existence. Many are happy to have come into being because they enjoy their lives. But these appraisals are mistaken for precisely the reasons I have outlined. The fact that one enjoys one's life does not make one's existence better than non-existence, because if one had not come into existence there would have been nobody to have missed the joy of leading that life and thus the absence of joy would not be bad. Notice, by contrast, that it makes sense to regret having come into existence if one does not enjoy one's life. In this case, if one had not come into existence then no being would have suffered the life one leads. That is good, even though there would be nobody who would have enjoyed that good.

Now it may be objected that one cannot possibly be mistaken about whether one's existence is preferable to non-existence. It might be said that just as one cannot be mistaken about whether one is in pain, one cannot be mistaken about whether one is glad to have been born. Thus if 'I am glad to have been born', a proposition to which many people would assent, is equivalent to 'It is better that I came into existence', then one cannot be mistaken about whether existence is better than non-existence. The problem with this line of reasoning is that these two propositions are not equivalent. Even if one cannot be mistaken about whether one *currently* is glad to have been born, it does not follow that one cannot be mistaken about whether it is better that one came into existence. We can imagine somebody being glad, at one stage in his life, that he came to be, and then (or earlier), perhaps in the midst of extreme agony, regretting his having come into existence. Now it cannot be the case that (all things considered) it is both better to have come into existence and better never to have come into existence. But that is exactly what we would have to say in such a case, if it were true that being glad or unhappy about having come into existence were equivalent to its actually being better or worse that one came into being. This is true even in those cases in which people do not change their minds about whether they are happy to have been born. Why so few people do change their minds is explained, at least in part, by the unduly rosy picture most people have about the quality of their own lives. In the coming chapter, I show that (with the exception of real pessimists, who may have an accurate view of how bad their lives are) people's lives are much worse than they think.

3

How Bad Is Coming into Existence?

> You may look upon life as an unprofitable episode, disturbing the blessed calm of non-existence.
>
> Arthur Schopenhauer[1]

> The fact of having been born is a very bad augury for immortality.
>
> George Santayana[2]

I have argued that so long as a life contains even the smallest quantity of bad, coming into existence is a harm. Whether or not one accepts this conclusion, one can recognize that a life containing a significant amount of bad is a harm. I turn now to show that all human lives contain much more bad than is ordinarily recognized. If people realized just how bad their lives were, they might grant that their coming into existence was a harm even if they deny that coming into existence would have been a harm had their lives contained but the smallest amount of bad. Thus this chapter can

---

[1] Schopenhauer, Arthur, 'On the Sufferings of the World', in *Complete Essays of Schopenhauer*, trans. T. Bailey Saunders, 5 (New York: Willey Book Company, 1942) 4.

[2] Santayana, George, *Reason in Religion* (vol. iii of *The Life of Reason*) (New York: Charles Scribner's Sons, 1922) 240.

be seen as providing a basis, independent of asymmetry and its implications, for regretting one's existence and for taking all actual cases of coming into existence to be harmful.

However, the arguments in this chapter can also be seen as a continuation of the argument in Chapter 2. The conclusion that coming into existence is *always* a harm tells us nothing about the *magnitude* of that harm. In the current chapter I consider the question of *how* bad it is to come into existence. The answer to this question depends on how bad the resultant life is. Even though everybody is harmed by being brought into existence, not all lives are equally bad. Thus, coming into existence will be a greater harm for some than for others. The worse a life is, the greater the harm of being brought into existence. I shall argue, however, that even the best lives are very bad, and therefore that being brought into existence is always a considerable harm. To clarify, I shall not be arguing that all lives are so bad that they are not worth continuing. That is a much stronger claim than I need to make. Instead, I shall be arguing that people's lives are much worse than they think and that all lives contain a great deal of bad.

WHY LIFE'S QUALITY
IS NOT THE DIFFERENCE
BETWEEN ITS GOOD AND ITS BAD

Many will be tempted to assess the quality of a life simply by subtracting the disvalue of life's negative features from the value of its positive features. That is to say, they will assign values to quadrants (1) and (2) in my schema, and then subtract the latter from the former.[3] However, this way of determining a life's quality is far too simplistic. How well or badly a life goes depends not simply on

---

[3] That the resultant number may sometimes be positive does not indicate, as I showed in Chapter 2, that existence is better than non-existence.

how much good and bad there is, but also on other considerations—most prominently considerations about how that good and bad is distributed.

One such consideration is the *order* of the good and bad. For instance, a life in which all the good occurred in the first half, and uninterrupted bad characterized the second half, would be a lot worse than one in which the good and bad were more evenly distributed. This is true even if the total amount of good and bad were the same in each life. Similarly, a life of steadily inclining achievement and satisfaction is preferable to one that starts out bright in the very earliest years but gets progressively worse.[4] The amount of good and bad in each of these alternative lives may be the same, but the trajectory can make one life better than the other.

Another distributional consideration is the *intensity* of the good and the bad. A life in which the pleasures were extraordinarily intense but correspondingly few, infrequent, and short-lived might be worse than a life with the same total amount of pleasure, but where the individual pleasures were less intense and more frequently distributed across the life. However, pleasures and other goods can also be distributed *too* widely within a life, thereby making them so mild as to be barely distinguishable from neutral states. A life so characterized might be worse than one in which there were a few more noticeable 'highs'.

A third way in which the distribution of good and bad within a life can affect that life's quality derives from the *length of life*. To be sure, the length of a life will interact dynamically with the quantity of good and bad. A long life with very little good would have to be characterized by significant quantities of bad, if only because the absence of sufficient good over such long periods would create tedium—a bad. Nevertheless, we can imagine lives of somewhat

---

[4] I am reminded of the (apocryphal?) story of a child who, having overachieved in primary school, was welcomed by the principal of his new high school with the following remark: 'I see that you have a great future behind you.'

unequal length that share the same quantity of good and of bad. One life might have more neutral features, sufficiently evenly distributed over the life not to affect the quantity of good or bad. In such cases, one might plausibly judge the longer life to be better (if the life is of sufficient quality to be worth continuing) or worse (if it is not).

There is a further (non-distributional) consideration that can affect an assessment of a life's quality. Arguably, once a life reaches a certain *threshold* of badness (considering both the amount and the distribution of its badness), no quantity of good can outweigh it, because no amount of good could be worth that badness.[5] It is just this assessment that Donald ('Dax') Cowart made of his own life—or at least of that part of his life following a gas explosion that burnt two-thirds of his body. He refused extremely painful, life-saving treatment, but the doctors ignored his wishes and treated him nonetheless. His life was saved, he achieved considerable success, and he reattained a satisfactory quality of life. Yet, he continued to maintain that these post-burn goods were not worth the costs of enduring the treatments to which he was subjected.[6] No matter how much good followed his recovery, this could not outweigh, at least in his own assessment, the bad of the burns and treatment that he experienced.

This point may be expressed more generally. Compare two lives—those of X and Y—and consider, for simplicity's sake, only the amount of good and bad (and not also the distributional considerations). X's life has (relatively) modest quantities of good and bad—perhaps fifteen kilo-units of positive value and five kilo-units of negative value. Y's life, by contrast, has unbearable quantities of bad (say, fifty kilo-units of negative value). Y's life also

---

[5] Instead of thresholds, Derek Parfit speaks of compensated and uncompensated suffering. (*Reasons and Persons*, 408.) Suffering is of one or other kind, depending on whether it is found in a life that is worth living.

[6] See, for example, Pence, Gregory E., *Classic Cases in Medical Ethics*, 2nd edn. (New York, McGraw-Hill, 1995) 54, 61.

has much more good (seventy kilo-units of positive value) than does X's. Nevertheless, X's life might reasonably be judged less bad, even if Y's has greater net value, judged in strictly quantitative terms—ten kilo-units versus twenty kilo-units of positive value. This shows further why the assignment of values in Figure 2.4 (in the previous chapter) must, as I argued there, be wrong.

From the foregoing reflections, it should be apparent that an assessment of how bad a life is must be more complicated than simply subtracting the good from the bad. It will not do, therefore, to attempt to calculate how bad a life is simply by subtracting the value of quadrant (2) from the value of quadrant (1).

WHY SELF-ASSESSMENTS OF ONE'S LIFE'S QUALITY ARE UNRELIABLE

Most people deny that their lives, all things considered, are bad (and they certainly deny that their lives are so bad as to make never existing preferable). Indeed, most people think that their lives go quite well. Such widespread blithe self-assessments of well-being, it is often thought, constitute a refutation of the view that life is bad. How, it is asked, can life be bad if most of those who live it deny that it is? How can it be a harm to come into existence if most of those who have come into existence are pleased that they did?

In fact, however, there is very good reason to doubt that these self-assessments are a reliable indicator of a life's quality. There are a number of well-known features of human psychology that can account for the favourable assessment people usually make of their own life's quality. It is these psychological phenomena rather than the actual quality of a life that explain (the extent of) the positive assessment.

The first, most general and most influential of these psychological phenomena is what some have called the Pollyanna Principle,[7] a

[7] Matlin, Margaret W., and Stang, David J., *The Pollyanna Principle: Selectivity in Language, Memory and Thought* (Cambridge MA: Schenkman Publishing Company,

tendency towards optimism.[8] This manifests in many ways. First, there is an inclination to recall positive rather than negative experiences. For example, when asked to recall events from throughout their lives, subjects in a number of studies listed a much greater number of positive than negative experiences.[9] This selective recall distorts our judgement of how well our lives have gone so far. It is not only assessments of our past that are biased, but also our projections or expectations about the future. We tend to have an exaggerated view of how good things will be.[10] The Pollyannaism typical of recall and projection is also characteristic of subjective judgements about current and overall well-being. Many studies have consistently shown that self-assessments of well-being are markedly skewed toward the positive end of the spectrum.[11] For

1978). The principle is named, of course, after Pollyanna, the protagonist of Eleanor Porter's children's book of that name. (Porter, Eleanor H. *Pollyanna*, (London: George G. Harrap & Co. 1927).)

[8] This is also discussed at great length in Taylor, Shelley E., *Positive Illusions: Creative Self-Deception and the Healthy Mind* (New York: Basic Books, 1989). There is quite a bit of evidence that happier people with greater self-esteem tend to have a less realistic view of themselves. Those with a more realistic view tend either to be depressed or have low self-esteem or both. For a discussion of this see Taylor, Shelley E., and Brown, Jonathon D., 'Illusion and Well-Being: A Social Psychological Perspective on Mental Health', *Psychological Bulletin*, 103/2 (1998) 193–210.

[9] The literature on this topic is reviewed by Matlin, M., and Stang, D. *The Pollyanna Principle*, 141–4. See also Greenwald, Anthony G. 'The Totalitarian Ego: Fabrication and Revision of Personal History', *American Psychologist*, 35/7 (1980) 603–18.

[10] For a review of some of this research see Taylor, S., and Brown, J., 'Illusion and Well-Being: A Social Psychological Perspective on Mental Health', 196–7. See also Matlin, M., and Stang, D., *The Pollyanna Principle*, 160–6. For examples of the primary literature see Weinstein, Neil D., 'Unrealistic Optimism about Future Life Events', *Journal of Personality and Social Psychology*, 39/5 (1980) 806–20; Weinstein, Neil D., 'Why it Won't Happen to Me: Perceptions of Risk Factors and Susceptibility', *Health Psychology*, 3/5 (1984) 431–57. The latter study suggests that the optimism extends only to those aspects of one's health that are *perceived* to be controllable.

[11] Inglehart, Ronald. *Culture Shift in Advanced Industrial Society* (Princeton NJ: Princeton University Press, 1990) 218 ff; Andrews, Frank M., and Withey, Stephen B., *Social Indicators of Well-Being: Americans' Perspectives of Life Quality* (New York: Plenum Press, 1976) 207 ff, 376; For an overview of various studies see also Diener, Ed., Diener, Carol, 'Most People are Happy', *Psychological Science*, 7/3 (1996) 181–5; and Myers, David G., and Diener, Ed., 'The Pursuit of Happiness', *Scientific American*, 274/5 (1996) 70–2.

instance, very few people describe themselves as 'not too happy'. Instead, the overwhelming majority claims to be either 'pretty happy' or 'very happy'.[12] Indeed, most people believe that they are better off than most others or than the average person.[13]

Most of the factors that plausibly improve the quality of a person's life do not commensurately influence self-assessments of that quality (where they influence them at all). For example, although there is a correlation between people's own rankings of their health and their subjective assessments of well-being, objective assessments of people's health, judging by physical symptoms, are not as good a predictor of peoples' subjective evaluations of their well-being.[14] Even among those whose dissatisfaction with their health does lead to lower self-reported well-being, most report levels of satisfaction toward the positive end of the spectrum.[15] Within any given country,[16] the poor are nearly (but not quite) as happy as the rich are. Nor do education and occupation make *much* (even though they do make

[12] Campbell, Angus., Converse, Philip E., and Rodgers, Willard L., *The Quality of American Life* (New York: Russell Sage Foundation, 1976) 24–5.

[13] Matlin, M., and Stang, D. (*The Pollyanna Principle*, 146–7) cite a number of studies that reached this conclusion. See also Andrews, F. M., and Withey, S. B., *Social Indicators of Well-Being*, 334.

[14] Diener, Ed., Suh, Eunkook M., Lucas, Richard E., and Smith, Heidi L., 'Subjective Well-Being: Three Decades of Progress', *Psychological Bulletin*, 125/2, (1999) 287. See also, Breetvelt, I. S., and van Dam, F. S. A. M., 'Underreporting by Cancer Patients: the Case of Response Shift', *Social Science and Medicine*, 32/9 (1991) 981–7. According to some studies, the handicapped and retarded have just as much life satisfaction as normal persons (Cameron, Paul., Titus, Donna G., Kostin, John., and Kostin, Marilyn., 'The Life Satisfaction of Nonnormal Persons', *Journal of Consulting and Clinical Psychology*, 41 (1973) 207–14. Yerxa, Elizabeth J., and Baum, Susan, 'Engagement in Daily Occupations and Life-Satisfaction Among People with Spinal Cord Injuries', *The Occupational Therapy Journal of Research*, 6/5 (1986) 271–83).

[15] Mehnert, Thomas., Krauss, Herbert H., Nadler, Rosemary., and Boyd, Mary., 'Correlates of Life Satisfaction in Those with Disabling Conditions', *Rehabilitative Psychology*, 35/1 (1990) 3–17, and especially p. 9.

[16] Interestingly, self-assessments of happiness and life satisfaction do vary more considerably between different countries. But everywhere there is a tendency towards optimism. What varies is the degree of optimism. Inglehart, R., *Culture Shift in Advanced Industrial Society*, 243.

some) difference.[17] Although there is some disagreement about how much each of the above and other factors affect subjective assessments of well-being, it is clear that even the sorts of events that one would have thought would make people 'very unhappy' have this effect on only a very small proportion of people.[18]

Another well-known psychological phenomenon that makes our self-assessments of well-being unreliable and that explains some (but not all) of the Pollyannaism just mentioned is the phenomenon of what might be called adaptation, accommodation, or habituation. When a person's objective well-being takes a turn for the worse, there is, at first, a significant subjective dissatisfaction. However, there is a tendency then to adapt to the new situation and to adjust one's expectations accordingly.[19] Although there is some dispute about how much adaptation occurs and how the extent of the adaptation varies in different domains of life, there is agreement that adaptation does occur.[20] As a result, even if the subjective sense of well-being does not return to the

[17] Andrews, F., and Withey, S., *Social Indicators of Well-Being*, 138–9; Inglehart, R., *Culture Shift in Advanced Industrial Society*, 227–32. Where extra education does make a difference it may make people less happy. See, for example, Campbell, A., et al, *The Quality of American Life*, 487.

[18] For a review of the impact of various external factors on subjective assessments of well-being, see Diener, Ed., et al, 'Subjective Well-Being: Three Decades of Progress', 286–94.

[19] Campbell, A., et al, *The Quality of American Life*, 163–4, 485. Brickman, Philip., Coates, Dan., and Janoff-Bulman, Ronnie. 'Lottery Winners and Accident Victims: Is Happiness Relative?', *Journal of Personality and Social Psychology*, 36/8 (1978) 917–27. Headey, Bruce., and Wearing, Alexander. 'Personality, Life Events, and Subjective Well-Being: Toward a Dynamic Equilibrium Model', *Journal of Personality and Social Psychology*, 57/4 (1989) 731–9. Suh, Eunkook., Diener, Ed., and Fujita, Frank., 'Events and Subjective Well-Being: Only Recent Events Matter', *Journal of Personality and Social Psychology*, 70/5 (1996) 1091–102. For a recent review of the literature see Ed Diener, et al, 'Subjective Well-Being: Three Decades of Progress', 285–6.

[20] For example, although not denying the phenomenon of adaptation, Richard A. Easterlin thinks that the extent of adaptation is sometimes exaggerated. See his 'Explaining Happiness', *Proceedings of the National Academy of Sciences*, 100/19 (2003) 11176–83, and 'The Economics of Happiness', *Daedalus*, Spring 2004, 26–33. As an aside, it is interesting that Professor Easterlin makes the mistake of thinking that if adaptation were complete, well-being could not be improved and 'public policies aimed at making people better off by improving their social and economic conditions are fruitless' ('The Economics of Happiness', 27). But this presupposes that there is

original level, it comes closer towards it than one might think, and it comes closer in some domains than in others. Because the subjective sense of well-being tracks recent change in the level of well-being better than it tracks a person's actual level of well-being, it is an unreliable indicator of the latter.

A third psychological factor that affects self-assessments of well-being is an implicit comparison with the well-being of others.[21] It is not so much how well one's life goes as how well it goes in comparison with others that determines one's judgement about how well one's life is going. Thus self-assessments are a better indicator of the *comparative* rather than *actual* quality of one's life. One effect of this is that those negative features of life that are shared by everybody are inert in people's judgements about their own well-being. Since these features are very relevant, overlooking them leads to unreliable judgements.

Of these three psychological phenomena, it is only Pollyannaism that inclines people unequivocally towards more positive assessments of how well their life is going. We adapt not only to negative situations but also to positive ones, and we compare ourselves not only with those who are worse off but also with those who are better off than we are. However, given the force of Pollyannaism, both adaptation and comparison operate both from an optimistic baseline and under the influence of optimistic biases. For example, people are more prone to comparing themselves with those who are worse off than with those who are better off.[22] Thus, in the best cases, adaptation and comparison reinforce Pollyannaism. In the worst cases, they mitigate it but do not negate it entirely. When we do adapt to the good or compare ourselves

no difference between one's perceived (subjective) and actual (objective) level of well-being.

[21] See, for example, Wood, Joanne V., 'What is Social Comparison and How Should We Study it?', *Personality and Social Psychology Bulletin*, 22/5 (1996) 520–37.

[22] This is discussed by Brown, Jonathon D., and Dutton, Keith A., 'Truth and Consequences: the Costs and Benefits of Accurate Self-Knowledge', *Personality and Social Psychology Bulletin*, 21/12 (1995) 1292.

with those who are better off than ourselves, our self-assessments are less positive than they otherwise would be, but they do not usually cause them to become negative.

The above psychological phenomena are unsurprising from an evolutionary perspective.[23] They militate against suicide and in favour of reproduction. If our lives are quite as bad as I shall still suggest they are, and if people were prone to see this true quality of their lives for what it is, they might be much more inclined to kill themselves, or at least not to produce more such lives. Pessimism, then, tends not to be naturally selected.[24]

THREE VIEWS ABOUT THE QUALITY OF LIFE, AND WHY LIFE GOES BADLY ON ALL OF THEM

An influential taxonomy[25] distinguishes three kinds of theory about the quality of a life. According to *hedonistic* theories, a life goes well or badly depending on the extent to which it is characterized by positive or negative mental states—pleasure and pain (broadly construed). According to *desire-fulfilment* theories, the quality of a person's life is assessed in terms of the extent to which his desires are fulfilled. What is desired might include mental states, but it can also include states of the (external) world. According to *objective list* theories, the quality of a life is determined by the extent to which it is characterized by certain objective goods and bads. On objective list theories, some things are good for us irrespective of whether they bring pleasure in any given situation

[23] For much more on this see Tiger, Lionel, *Optimism: The Biology of Hope* (New York: Simon and Schuster, 1979).

[24] This is not to say that there is no limit on the degree of optimism that has an evolutionary advantage. Too much optimism can be maladaptive, and a certain amount of pessimism has its advantages. See, for example, Waller, Bruce N., 'The Sad Truth: Optimism, Pessimism and Pragmatism', in *Ratio* new series, 16 (2003) 189–97.

[25] Parfit, Derek, *Reasons and Persons*, 493–502.

and irrespective of whether we desire them. Other things are bad for us whether or not they bring pain and whether or not we desire them. Obviously objective list theories could differ from one another on the basis of the goods and bads on their lists. One author[26] suggests that the goods include accomplishment, the 'components of human existence' (including agency, basic capabilities, and liberty), understanding, enjoyment, and deep personal relations. Another author lists possible candidate goods as 'moral goodness, rational activity, the development of one's abilities, having children and being a good parent, knowledge, and the awareness of true beauty'.[27] This author suggests that among the bad things would be 'being betrayed, manipulated, slandered, deceived, being deprived of liberty or dignity, and enjoying either sadistic pleasure, or aesthetic pleasure in what is in fact ugly'.[28] Objective list theories are the most expansive of the three kinds of theory in that they can include some pleasures and the fulfilment of some desires, subject to the constraints of other features of the list.

To show how bad life is and therefore how bad it is to come into existence, it is not necessary to choose between hedonistic, desire-fulfilment, and objective list theories. Instead, it can be shown how life is very bad irrespective of which of these sorts of theory one adopts.

Hedonistic theories

Consider first the hedonistic view. Such a view will need to distinguish between three kinds of mental states—negative ones, positive ones, and neutral ones. Negative mental states include discomfort, pain, suffering, distress, guilt, shame, irritation, boredom, anxiety, frustration, stress, fear, grief, sadness, and loneliness. Positive mental states—pleasures, in the broad sense—can be of two kinds. First, there are those which are relief from

---

[26] Griffin, James, *Well-Being* (Oxford: Clarendon Press, 1986) 67.
[27] Parfit, Derek, *Reasons and Persons*, 499.   [28] Ibid.

negative mental states. These relief pleasures include the subsiding of a pain (such as a headache), the mollification of an itch, the abatement of boredom, the alleviation of stress, the dissipation of anxiety or fear, and the assuagement of guilt. Secondly, there are the intrinsically positive states. Intrinsic pleasures include pleasant sensory experiences—tastes, smells, visual images, sounds, and tactile sensations—as well as some non-sensory conscious states (such as joy, love, and excitement). Some pleasures have both relief and intrinsic components. For example, eating a tasty meal while hungry brings both relief from hunger and the intrinsic pleasure of fine-tasting food. (By contrast, eating insipid food while hungry might relieve the hunger, but it would do so without the intrinsic pleasure.[29]) Neutral mental states are those which are neither negative, nor positive in either the relief or intrinsic sense. Neutral states include the *absence* of pain, fear, or shame (as distinct from gaining *relief* from these negative states).

For the psychological reasons mentioned earlier, we tend to ignore just how much of our lives is characterized by negative mental states, even if often only relatively mildly negative ones. Consider, for example, conditions causing negative mental states daily or more often. These include hunger, thirst, bowel and bladder distension (as these organs become filled), tiredness, stress, thermal discomfort (that is, feeling either too hot or too cold), and itch. For billions of people, at least some of these discomforts are chronic. These people cannot relieve their hunger, escape the cold, or avoid the stress. However, even those who can find some relief do not do so immediately or perfectly, and thus experience them to some extent every day. In fact, if we think about it, significant periods of each day are marked by some or other of these states. For example, unless one is eating and drinking so regularly as to prevent hunger and thirst or countering them as they arise, one is likely hungry and thirsty for a few hours a day. Unless one is lying

---

[29] This is not to deny that food can taste better if one is hungry.

about all day, one is probably tired for a substantial portion of one's waking life. How often does one feel neither too hot nor too cold, but exactly right?[30]

Of course, we tend *not* to think about how much of our lives is marked by these states. The three psychological phenomena, outlined in the previous section, explain why this is so. Because of Pollyannaism we overlook the bad (and especially the relatively mildly bad). Adaptation also plays a role. People are *so* used to the discomforts of daily life that they overlook them entirely, even though they are so pervasive. Finally, since these discomforts are experienced by everybody else too, they do not serve to differentiate the quality of one's own life from the quality of the lives of others. The result is that normal discomforts are not detected on the radar of subjective assessment of well-being. That we do not think of how much of our daily lives are pervaded by the discomforts mentioned does not mean that our daily lives are not pervaded by them. That there is so much discomfort is surely relevant on the hedonistic view.

The negative mental states mentioned so far, however, are simply the baseline ones characteristic of *healthy* daily life. Chronic ailments and advancing age make matters worse. Aches, pains, lethargy, and sometimes frustration from disability become an experiential backdrop for everything else.

Now add those discomforts, pains, and sufferings that are experienced either less frequently or only by some (though nonetheless very many) people. These include allergies, headaches, frustration, irritation, colds, menstrual pains, hot flushes, nausea, hypoglycaemia, seizures, guilt, shame, boredom, sadness, depression, loneliness, body-image dissatisfaction, the ravages of AIDS, of cancer, and of other such life-threatening diseases, and grief and bereavement. The reach of negative mental states in ordinary lives is extensive.

---

[30] The Goldilocks condition!

This is not to deny that there are also intrinsic pleasures in a life. These pleasures sometimes occur in the absence of negative mental states, and are best when they do. Intrinsic pleasures can also coexist with the negative ones (so long as the negative states are not of sufficient intensity to undo the pleasure entirely). Neutral states and relief pleasures obviously can also affect the quality of a life. It is better to have a neutral state than a negative one, and if one has a negative state, relief from it (as soon as possible) is better than no relief. Nevertheless, there would be something absurd about living *for* neutral states or relief pleasures, or about starting a life in order to create more neutral conscious states or to produce more relief pleasure. Neutral states and relief pleasures can be valuable only in so far as they displace negative states. The argument that it is better never to come into existence explains why it is also absurd to start a life for the *intrinsic* pleasures that that life will contain. The reason for this is that even the intrinsic pleasures of existing do not constitute a net benefit over never existing. Once alive, it is good to have them, but they are purchased at the cost of life's misfortune—a cost that is quite considerable.

Desire-fulfilment theories

The foregoing is relevant to assessing the quality of a life not only on a hedonistic view but also on a desire-fulfilment view. This is because many of our desires are for positive mental states and the absence of negative ones. Given just how many negative mental states we have, the many desires for their absence are thwarted. We also desire pleasures and *some* of those desires are satisfied. However, as I shall show, there is a lot of dissatisfaction and not that much satisfaction, contrary to what many people think.

Notwithstanding the overlap between hedonistic and desire-fulfilment theories, there is a clear difference between them. This is because there can be positive mental states in the absence of fulfilled desires, and there can be fulfilled desires in the absence of positive mental states. The former can occur when

a) one mistakenly believes that a desire has been fulfilled; or
b) one finds that one did not need the desire fulfilled in order to attain the positive mental state.

The latter can occur when

a) one mistakenly believes that a desire has not been fulfilled; or
b) one's desire was not for a positive mental state and the satisfaction of the desire does not bring about such a state; or
c) one finds that the fulfilled desire did not produce the positive mental state one thought it would.

In all such cases desire-fulfilment theories require us to judge the quality of a person's life on the basis of whether the desires were or were not fulfilled and not on the basis of whether or not one had pleasant mental states.

Although one can be mistaken about how much of one's life has or will be characterized by positive mental states, one cannot be mistaken about whether one is, right now, experiencing a positive or a negative mental state. With desires, however, the scope for error is arguably greater because one *can* be mistaken right now about whether one's desires have been fulfilled (unless those desires are for pleasures). Thus we have less privileged access to whether our desires have been satisfied. This introduces further scope for error in self-assessments of well-being. Given Pollyannaism, it is evident that this error will tend towards *over*estimation of how good life is on the desire-fulfilment view.

Rather little of our lives is characterized by satisfied desires and rather a lot is marked by unsatisfied desires. Consider first how vulnerable our desires are to the vicissitudes of life. No desires for that which we lack are ever satisfied immediately. Such a desire must be present *before* it can be satisfied and thus we endure a period of frustration before the desire is fulfilled. It is logically possible for desires to be fulfilled very soon after they arise, but given the way the world is, this does not usually happen. Instead, we usually persist in a state of desire for a period of time. This time may vary—from minutes to decades. As I said before, one usually waits at least a couple of hours until hunger is satiated (unless one is on a 'hunger-prevention' or a 'nip-hunger-in-the-bud' diet). One waits still longer to get rest when one is tired. Children wait years to gain independence. Adolescents and adults can wait years to fulfil desires for personal satisfaction or professional success. Where one's desires are fulfilled, this fulfilment is often ephemeral. One desires public office and is elected but not re-elected. One's desire to be married is eventually fulfilled, but then one gets divorced. One wants a holiday but it ends (too soon). Often one's desires are never fulfilled. One yearns to be free, but dies incarcerated or oppressed. One seeks wisdom but never attains it. One hankers after being beautiful but is congenitally and irreversibly ugly. One aspires to great wealth and influence, but remains poor and impotent all one's life. One has a desire not to believe falsehoods, but unknowingly clings to such beliefs all one's life. Very few people ever attain the kind of control over their lives and circumstances that they would like.

Not all one's desires are for that which one lacks. Sometimes we desire not to lose that which we already have. Such desires, by definition, have immediate satisfaction, but the sad truth is that that fulfilment often does not last. One has a desire not to lose one's health and youth, but it happens all too quickly. The wrinkles appear, the hair goes grey or falls out, the back aches, arthritis ravages one's joints, the eyes weaken, one becomes flabby and saggy. One wishes not to be bereaved, but unless one's desire not to die is thwarted sooner rather than later, one must soon face the death of grandparents, parents, and other dear ones.

As if this were not bad enough, consider next what we might call the 'treadmill of desires'. Although the fulfilment of some desires is temporary because the fulfilment becomes undone, desire fulfilment is much more often temporary because even though the desire remains fulfilled another desire arises in its place. Thus the initial satisfaction soon gives way to new desires.

Among the psychologists who have recognized this is Abraham Maslow, who famously observed a hierarchy of needs. (Although there is a difference between needs and desires, they both have the same feature I am discussing here.) Professor Maslow noted that

need gratifications lead only to temporary happiness which in turn tends to be succeeded by another and (hopefully) higher discontent. It looks as if the human hope for eternal happiness can never be fulfilled. Certainly happiness does come and is obtainable and is real. But it looks as if we must accept its intrinsic transience, especially if we focus on its more intense forms.[31]

And Ronald Inglehart noted that if getting what we wanted made us lastingly happy, we would no longer engage in goal-pursuing activities.[32] Subjective well-being, he said, 'reflects a balance between one's aspirations and one's situation—and with long term prosperity, one's aspirations tend to rise, adjusting to the situation'.[33]

Abraham Maslow writes disapprovingly of our perpetual discontent.[34] By contrast, the great philosophical pessimist Arthur Schopenhauer, who much earlier noted this fact of life, took it to be inevitable.[35] Life, on the Schopenhauerian view, is a constant state of striving or willing—a state of dissatisfaction. Attaining that for which one strives brings a transient satisfaction, which

[31] Maslow, Abraham, *Motivation and Personality* 2nd edn. (New York: Harper & Row Publishers, 1970) p. xv.

[32] Inglehart, R., *Culture Shift in Advanced Industrial Society*, 212.

[33] Ibid.

[34] He refers to the observation that we have this feature as 'Grumble Theory' (*Motivation and Personality*, p. xv). He refers to one's 'failing to count one's blessings' as 'not realistic and can therefore be considered to be a form of pathology' which, he says, can in 'most instances be cured very easily, simply by experiencing the appropriate deprivation or lack' (p. 61).

[35] See, for example, Schopenhauer, Arthur, *The World as Will and Representation*, trans. E. F. J. Payne (New York: Dover Publications, 1966) 318, 362.

soon yields to some new desire. Were striving to end, the result would be boredom, another kind of dissatisfaction.[36] Striving is thus an unavoidable part of life. We cease striving only when we cease living.

Arthur Schopenhauer would also have rejected Professor Maslow's claim that happiness is real. On the Schopenhauerian view, suffering is all that exists independently.[37] Happiness, for him, is but a temporary absence of suffering. Satisfaction is the ephemeral fulfilment of desire. In hedonistic terms, there are no intrinsic pleasures. All pleasures are simply passing relief from negative mental states.

One need not reject, as Arthur Schopenhauer does, the independent existence of happiness to accept his view that suffering is endemic to and pervasive in life. Fulfilled desires, like pleasures (even of the intrinsic kind), are states of achievement rather than default states. For instance, one has to work at satiating oneself, while hunger comes naturally. After one has eaten or taken liquid, bowel and bladder discomfort ensues quite naturally and we have to seek relief. One has to seek out pleasurable sensations, in the absence of which blandness comes naturally. The upshot of this is that we must continually work at keeping suffering (including tedium) at bay, and we can do so only imperfectly. Dissatisfaction does and must pervade life. There are moments, perhaps even periods, of satisfaction, but they occur against a background of dissatisfied striving. Pollyannaism may cause most people to blur out this background, but it remains there.

Now it may be objected that the foregoing makes matters sound worse than they really are. Although our desires are not fulfilled immediately and although a fulfilled desire gives way to a new desire, the period during which the desire is unfulfilled and during which we may strive towards its fulfilment is valuable. There

---

[36] Ibid. 312.
[37] Schopenhauer, Arthur, 'On the Sufferings of the World', in *Complete Essays of Schopenhauer,* trans. T. Bailey Saunders, 5 (New York: Willey Book Company, 1942) 1.

is something positive either in the striving or in the period of deprivation, or both.

There are two ways of making sense of this objection on a desire-fulfilment view. The first is to say that in addition to desiring whatever we desire, we desire striving to fulfil that desire. Thus the striving fulfils a desire on the way to fulfilling another desire. As a result our desires are not as unsatisfied as I have suggested they are. The second way of making sense of the objection is to say that whether or not we desire the period of deprivation or the striving to fulfil our (other) desires, such a precursor to desire fulfilment makes the eventual fulfilment that much sweeter.

On both of these interpretations the objection has its limitations. I concede that some people do enjoy the process of fulfilling some desires. There surely are some writers, for example, who enjoy the process of writing a poem or a book, and some gardeners may enjoy the process of growing the desired vegetables. However, it is probably the case that Pollyannaism and the other psychological features cause more people either to think that they desire the process or not to mind having the desire unfulfilled during it. Notwithstanding these psychological features, not everybody desires the process of fulfilling a desire. Some writers may loathe the creative process and enjoy only *having* produced a poem or a book. Some gardeners may hate gardening but do it only in order to be able to eat. Moreover, there are some desires the striving to which *nobody* could (reasonably) desire. Consider, for example, the process of fighting cancer. One wants to be cured of cancer but who actually wants to fight the battle, enduring the treatment and side-effects, and not knowing, along the way, whether it will be successful?

It is often more plausible to say that the value of not having desires fulfilled immediately is that the period of deprivation and the process of working towards fulfilment enhances the satisfaction when the desire is eventually fulfilled. We enjoy food more when we eat while hungry than we do when we eat while satiated.

Winning a race is a greater satisfaction when one has trained hard. One feels more satisfied to attain the goal of playing a complicated piece of music if one has had to work long hours to master it.

Again it is noteworthy that this cannot be said of all desires. But even among those desires of which it is true, for at least some of them it would be better, all things considered, if no striving were necessary. Freedom may be valued more if it were long desired or the result of a protracted struggle, but it would still be better not to have been deprived of freedom all that time. Long incarceration followed by freedom simply is not better than lifelong freedom. In other words, we must not mistakenly think that the redeeming features of deprivation and striving are actually advantages over more rapid desire fulfilment.

It might be thought that this applies to relatively few desires, but whatever may be true of the actual world, we can imagine a world in which we were differently constituted such that a period of deprivation and striving were unnecessary. Some people say that they cannot imagine such a world, but this is simply a failure of imagination. For example, as we are currently constituted, being hungry for a few hours enhances a meal. We can imagine beings that must be hungry for days in order to attain the same effect. Surely they are worse off than we are because their desires must remain unsatisfied for longer before they can gain the same satisfaction. But we are similarly worse off than we would be if we did not have to get as hungry as we do have to get in order to attain the same level of satisfaction from a meal. In other words, to show that we require the period of deprivation and striving to gain the most from the eventual fulfilment of the desire is not to show that our lives are better for that deprivation and striving. Instead it is to concede an unfortunate fact about our lives. It simply would be better if desire fulfilment required less unfulfilment along the way.

So far I have discussed how much unfulfilment characterizes life. I turn now to show that people overestimate the significance of that fulfilment that does exist. In other words, if we understand why our desires *are* fulfilled to the extent they are, we are left with a still grimmer picture.

On desire-fulfilment views, our lives go well to the extent that our desires are satisfied. However, the state of having one's desires fulfilled can be attained in one of two ways:

(a) having fulfilled whatever desires one has, or
(b) having only those desires that will be fulfilled.[38]

A crude desire-fulfilment view will not distinguish between these two ways of having one's desires fulfilled. The problem with such a crude view is that a terrible life could be transformed into a splendid one by expunging desires or by altering what one desires. If, for instance, one came to desire the various features of one's doleful existence, one's life would thereby transmute from the miserable to the magnificent. This is hard to swallow. It might *seem* (or feel) as though one's life had so improved, but it surely would not actually have been so transformed (even though it would actually have improved in a more limited way by feeling better).

The question is whether a more plausible version of a desire-fulfilment view can be constructed—one that judges a life to go better when desire-fulfilment is attained via (a) rather than (b). As this is a problem internal to desire-fulfilment theory, I shall not pursue this question. Suffice it to say that if such a version of the desire-fulfilment view cannot be formulated, then so much the worse for the desire-fulfilment view. But what if such a version could be constructed? We would then need to notice that because of the psychological phenomena I have outlined, (b) would account for much of our desire-fulfilment. Our desires are formulated and shaped in response to the limits of our situation. Therefore, our lives are much worse than they would be if our desire-fulfilment were exclusively (or even primarily) attributable to (a).

---

[38] Alternatively, the distinction might be expressed negatively by noting that there are two ways of not having one's desires frustrated: a) not having frustrated whatever desires one has; or b) not having desires (that will be frustrated).

There are those, such as Buddhists and Stoics, who believe that expunging or altering desires is exactly what we should be doing.[39] Believing this, however, is different from believing that (b) is preferable to (a). Indeed, recommending (b) is most reasonable as a response to the *impossibility* of (a).[40] In other words, (a) would be better and we must resort to (b) only because we cannot have (a). Acknowledging this does not undermine the view that our lives are much worse under (b) than they would be under (a).

Objective list theories

The discussions of hedonistic and desire-fulfilment views apply also to objective list views. Pleasurable mental states and the absence of painful ones must be on the list of objective goods. Similarly, the list of objective goods must include the fulfilment of some desires. Moreover, just as our desires adapt to our circumstances and are formulated by comparing ourselves with others, so objective lists of life's goods are constructed in a way that makes it possible for at least some people to be said to flourish. That is to say, 'objective lists' of goods are not constructed *sub specie aeternitatis*—from a truly objective perspective. Instead they are constructed *sub specie humanitatis*—from a human perspective. Unlike desires, which can vary from individual to individual, objective lists tend to apply to all people, or at least to whole classes or groups of people. They are taken to be objective only in the sense that they do not vary from

[39] The highest state of being, on the Buddhist view, is nirvana, a state in which all desire and (thus) all earthly suffering has been expunged. Whereas Buddhists think that this state can be attained during life, Arthur Schopenhauer would deny this, and I would agree with him. However, Buddhists do think that attaining the state of nirvana enables one to escape the cycle of reincarnation. In this sense the Buddhist view comes closer to the Schopenhauerian view—the end of desiring is connected with the end of (embodied) life.

[40] This is not to deny that it is preferable to expunge *some* desires—on moral or aesthetic grounds, perhaps. In these cases, however, the reason for expunging the desire is not that it cannot be fulfilled but that it would be inappropriate to fulfil it.

person to person. They are not taken to be objective in the sense of judging what a good life is *sub specie aeternitatis*.

Constructing lists *sub specie humanitatis* would be reasonable if one wanted to determine how well a particular life goes *in comparison* with other (human) lives. But knowing how well a particular life goes in comparison with other lives tells us very little about the baseline—how good human life is. If one's aim is to determine how good human life is, then the human perspective, given the psychological phenomena mentioned earlier, is manifestly an unreliable perspective from which to decide on what should be on the list of goods. From the human perspective, what we take to be worthwhile is very much determined by the limits of what we can expect.

For instance, since none of us lives until age 240, people tend not to think that failing to reach that age makes one's life go less well. However, most people regard it as tragic when somebody dies at forty (at least if that person's quality of life was comparatively good). But why should a death at ninety not be tragic if a death at forty is? The only answer can be that our judgement is constrained by our circumstances. We do not take that which is beyond our reach as something that would be a crucial good. But why must it be that the good life is within our reach? Perhaps the good life is something that is impossible to attain. It certainly sounds as though a life that is devoid of any discomfort, pain, suffering, distress, stress, anxiety, frustration, and boredom, that lasts for much longer than ninety years, and that is filled with much more of what is good would be better than the sort of life the luckiest humans have. Why then do we not judge our lives in terms of that (impossible) standard?

Or consider the meaning of life. A very plausible candidate for the list of objective goods is a life's having meaning. A meaningless life would be lacking an important good, even if it had other goods. Many people do think, even if only occasionally, that all lives lack meaning. They look at life *sub specie aeternitatis* and see no point to it. Conscious life, although but a blip on the radar of cosmic time, is laden with suffering—suffering that is directed to no end other than its own perpetuation. Most people, however, find the idea of life's meaninglessness intolerable and suggest that our lives *are* meaningful. Many (but not all) of these resort to a different perspective—that of humanity or that of an individual person—from which at least some lives can be meaningful. A life devoted to the service of humanity, for example, can be meaningful, *sub specie humanitatis*, even if, from the perspective of the universe, it is not. Other lives, though, such as that of the man who devotes his life to counting the number of blades of grass on different lawns,[41] would lack meaning *sub specie humanitatis*. The grass-counter's life could be meaningful, however, from his own subjective perspective, if he derived satisfaction from his unusual life's project. That his life could be meaningful from this perspective leads many people to think that the subjective perspective is unsatisfactory. But why should we think that the perspective of humanity is any more reliable than the perspective of the individual? From the perspective of the universe, the lives of both the philanthropist and the grass-counter are meaningless (which is not to say that philanthropy is not better than grass counting).

Some argue that it does not matter that our lives are meaningless from the perspective of the universe. Even if that were true, it would surely be much better if our lives had meaning independently of our own human perspective—if they mattered from the perspective of the universe. Thus, at the very least, we should see that our lives are much less good for not mattering from that perspective. Add to this the recognition of Pollyannaism and the other distorting psychological phenomena, and we have good reason for thinking that we may be overestimating how good our lives are by having meaning only from the perspective of humanity. It may

---

[41] The example is John Rawls's.

very well be that an important kind of meaning is impossible and that our lives are lacking an important good.

Against my argument that human lives are seriously wanting when judged *sub specie aeternitatis*, two objections may be raised. The first comes from those who say that they simply cannot imagine this perspective and thus cannot judge human lives from it. For example, they cannot imagine what a much longer life devoid of pain and frustration, and characterized by much greater wisdom, knowledge, and understanding would be like. This objection can be met in the same way that I met a similar objection to my comments on life's quality under the desire-fulfilment view. That is, I reject it as a failure of imagination. Perhaps we are not able to imagine, for example, exactly what it would feel like to be much more cognitively sophisticated than humans are. Nevertheless we can draw on our understanding of the differences between children and adults, and between animals and humans, to understand what kind of difference increased cognitive capacity would make. In this particular case there is room for debate about whether it would make our lives better. Whether it would depends in part on whether one thinks that our cognitive edge makes our lives better than cognitively less sophisticated animals. Humans are inclined to answer the latter question affirmatively, but that is not obviously the right answer. Understanding carries many costs. If one thinks that our extra cognition nonetheless makes our lives richer or better than those of non-human primates, we must concede that it would be still better if we were better equipped cognitively. That is unless we can show that we have the ideal degree of cognitive ability, which sounds suspiciously self-serving. If, by contrast, we think that we are worse off than non-human primates on account of our heightened cognitive abilities, then this is a further way in which our lives are worse than they could be.

There is a second, more compelling objection to my argument. This is the objection that judgements of quality of life *must* be context specific. A suitable analogy is that of a teacher marking a student's essay or exam.[42] What standard does the teacher set? If the pupils are twelve years old, the teacher must surely set the standard at a level suitable to twelve-year olds (and perhaps, more specifically, to those twelve-year olds). A twelve-year old's academic performance cannot be judged by standards suitable for postgraduate university students. Similarly, the objection goes, we must judge the quality of a human life by human standards and not *sub specie aeternitatis*.

Clearly, I do not deny that the work of twelve-year olds should be judged by standards suitable to their age. This is because in judging the work of a twelve-year old, we want to know how he or she compares with others in the same class. There are analogous purposes in sometimes adopting a human standard for judging the quality of human lives. We might want to know how well one human's life goes relative to the lives of other humans. Such comparisons have their value, but they are not the only way of making assessments.

To this it might be replied that just as we never then switch to a higher standard when assessing a twelve-year old child's work, we should never switch to a supra-human perspective to judge the quality of a human life. But there are a number of problems with this reply. For instance, we are never in danger of thinking that simply because a twelve-year old gets an 'A' by standards suitable for twelve-year olds that that child should be offered a chair of Physics at a prestigious university. That is to say, we have a clear understanding that the standard we are using is one suited to a twelve-year old, but that there are clear limits on that child's level of understanding. Yet people do regularly think that because some people's lives go well by human standards that they go as well as one could imagine.

At this point my interlocutor might offer the rejoinder that just as we never judge Physics professors by supra-human standards

---

[42] I am grateful to Andy Altman for this objection and analogy.

of intellect, so we should not judge the best human lives by supra-human standards of quality. The problem, though, is that we sometimes do and should judge the brightest people by supra-human standards. This becomes evident if we consider the philosophical problem of modesty (about one's attributes or achievements). This problem is that it is hard to explain what modesty is without undermining the case for its being understood as a virtue. If, for example, the modest person is understood as one who does not recognize that he has some superlative attribute, then modesty is an epistemic shortcoming and it is hard to see that as a virtue. If the modest person is one who knows how good he is but acts as though he does not, then modesty is a form of deception, which is an implausible candidate for a virtue. The best solution to the problem of modesty is to say that although the modest person has an accurate perception of his strengths, he also recognizes that there is a higher standard by which he falls short.[43] His ability to see himself *sub specie aeternitatis* puts his attributes and achievements in a perspective that makes him modest. It is this that we take to be a virtue.

I am recommending a more 'modest' view of the quality of the best human lives. I grant that it may sometimes be appropriate—when one is discussing distributive justice, for example—to compare the quality of some human lives with others. On other occasions, however, it is more appropriate to assess human lives *sub specie aeternitatis*. That is just the case when we wish to determine how good human life in general is. The quality of human life is then found wanting.

---

[43] This view is advanced by Richards, Norvin, 'Is Humility a Virtue?', *American Philosophical Quarterly*, 25/3 (1988) 253–9. Professor Richards does not suggest, as I shall now do, that the higher standard is the perspective of the universe. However, that standard makes the explanation of modesty most plausible—for otherwise modesty would be impossible for those who are literally the best humans in some area.

Concluding comments about the three views

All three views I have examined—the hedonistic view, the desire-fulfilment view and the objective list view—all allow a distinction between

a) how good a person's life actually is, and
b) how good it is thought to be.

Some people have a difficulty in seeing how this distinction is possible under the hedonistic view. They think that because a hedonistic view is about subjective mental states a person's subjective assessment of his quality of life must be reliable. However, the hedonistic view says that life is better or worse to the extent that it is *actually* characterized by positive or negative mental states. Since people can be mistaken about that, the hedonistic view does indeed allow the distinction between (a) and (b).

This is not to deny that (a) and (b) interact. If one's life is very bad, on any one of the three views, and one thinks that it is not, then in this one way it is actually better than it would be if one realized how bad it actually was. But to say that it is better in this way is neither to say that it is better in every way, nor is it to say that it is so much better that it is as good as one thinks it is.

I have argued that the quality of people's lives is much worse than they think, and I have shown how an understanding of human psychology can explain why people think that their lives are better than they really are. With a more accurate picture of the quality of an ordinary human life, we are in a better position to determine whether starting such a life is indecent, given that starting a new life can never benefit the person whose life is begun. Questions of decency and indecency are notoriously hard to answer, of course. However, if we employ a quite reasonable test, we find that it must indeed be indecent to start lives that are filled with as much harm as characterizes ordinary human lives.

The test is this: ask whether the amount of harm in a life could decently be inflicted on an already existent being, but neither to advance that being's overall interests nor for utilitarian purposes. The first condition—excluding that person's own interests—is obviously crucial given the argument that coming into existence can never be a benefit to the person who comes into existence. The second condition may be thought to be more controversial. However, it should not be. I have already argued that the most plausible versions of utilitarianism do not favour the creation of new people.[44] Creating new people does bring benefits to people other than the person created, but these are modest benefits to other individuals (to be discussed in Chapter 4) rather than the maximizing benefits of utilitarianism.

I have not argued, nor need I have argued, that all lives are so bad that they are not worth continuing. I have argued instead that all lives contain substantial amounts of whatever is thought bad. As I argued earlier in this chapter, determining the quality of a person's life is not simply a matter of determining how much good and bad there is in a life. Nevertheless, if a life contains more bad than one thinks, one's assessment of that life's quality cannot become more favourable. My arguments in Chapter 2 showed that even lesser quantities of bad could not be outweighed by whatever limited good a life may contain.

A WORLD OF SUFFERING

Such is the strength of Pollyannaism, that the foregoing sort of pessimism is often dismissed as the self-pitying whinging of existential weaklings. Optimists make valiant attempts to paint a rosy picture, to put a redeeming positive gloss on the human predicament, or at

[44] In Chapter 6 I shall consider the question whether any theoretical approach could permit temporary and highly limited baby-making as a means to phased extinction.

least to show a brave face. Pessimists find these unseemly—akin to jocularity or cheering at a funeral. Arthur Schopenhauer, for example, says of optimism that 'where it is not merely the thoughtless talk of those who harbour nothing but words under their shallow foreheads, seems to. . .be not merely an absurd, but also a really *wicked*, way of thinking, a bitter mockery of the unspeakable suffering of mankind'.[45]

Whether or not one accepts the pessimistic view I have presented of ordinary healthy life, the optimist is surely on very weak ground when one considers the amount of unequivocal suffering the world contains.[46] (I shall focus here only on *human* suffering, but the picture becomes still more obscene when we consider the suffering of the trillions of animals who share our planet—including the billions who are brought into existence each year, only to be maltreated and killed for human consumption or other use.)

Consider first, natural disasters. More than fifteen million people are thought to have died from such disasters in the last 1,000 years.[47] In the last few years, flooding, for example, has killed an estimated 20,000 annually and brought suffering to 'tens of millions'.[48] The number is greater in some years. In late December 2004, a few hundred thousand people lost their lives in a tsunami.

Approximately 20,000 people die every *day* from hunger.[49] An estimated 840 million people suffer from hunger and malnutrition

---

[45] Schopenhauer, Arthur, *The World as Will and Representation*, 326.

[46] Arthur Schopenhauer says:

If we were to conduct the most hardened and callous optimist through hospitals, infirmaries, operating theatres, through prisons, torture-chambers, and slave hovels, over battlefields and to places of execution; if we were to open to him all the dark abodes of misery, where it shuns the gaze of cold curiosity, and finally were to allow him to glance into the dungeon of Ugolino where prisoners starved to death, he too would certainly see in the end what kind of a world is this *meilleur des mondes possibles* [best of all possible worlds]. Ibid. 325.

[47] McGuire, Bill, *A Guide to the End of the World* (New York: Oxford University Press, 2002) 31.

[48] Ibid. 5.

[49] The Hunger Project:<http://www.thp.org>(accessed November 2003).

without dying from it.[50] That is a sizeable proportion of the approximately 6.3 billion people who currently live.

Disease ravages and kills millions annually. Consider plague, for example. Between 541 CE and 1912, it is estimated that over 102 million people succumbed to plague.[51] Remember that the human population during this period was just a fraction of its current size. The 1918 influenza epidemic killed 50 million people. Given the size of the current world human population and the increased speed and volume of global travel, a new influenza epidemic could cause millions more deaths. HIV currently kills nearly 3 million people annually.[52] If we add all other infectious diseases, we get a total of nearly 11 million deaths per year,[53] preceded by considerable suffering. Malignant neoplasms take more than a further 7 million lives each year,[54] usually after considerable and often protracted suffering. Add the approximately 3.5 million accidental deaths (including over a million road accident deaths a year).[55] When all other deaths are added, a colossal sum of approximately 56.5 million people died in 2001.[56] That is more than 107 people per minute. As the world human population grows the number of deaths increases. In some parts of the world, where infant mortality is high, many of these deaths will follow within a few years of birth. However, even when life expectancy is greater, we know that more birth leads to more death. Now multiply the number of deaths by the number of family and friends who survive to mourn and miss the departed. For every death there are many more bereft who grieve for the deceased.

Although much disease is attributable to human behaviour, consider the more intentionally caused suffering that some members

[50] 'Undernourishment Around the World',<http://www.fao/org/DOCREP/005/y7352E/y7352e03.htm>(accessed 14 November 2003)

[51] Rummel, R. J., *Death by Government* (New Brunswick, Transaction Publishers, 1994) 70.

[52] World Health Organization, *The World Health Report 2002* (Geneva: WHO, 2002) 186. The number for 2001 was 2,866,000.

[53] Ibid. 186.   [54] Ibid. 188.

[55] These are 2001 statistics. *The World Health Report 2002*, 190.

[56] Ibid. 186

of our species inflict on others. One authority estimates that before the twentieth century over 133 million people were killed in mass killings.[57] According to this same author, the first 88 years of the twentieth century saw 170 million (and possibly as many as 360 million) people 'shot, beaten, tortured, knifed, burned, starved, frozen, crushed, or worked to death; buried alive, drowned,. . .[hanged], bombed, or killed in any other of the myriad ways governments have inflicted death on unarmed, helpless citizens and foreigners'.[58]

Millions of people, obviously, are killed during wars. According to the *World Report on Violence and Health*, there were 1.6 million conflict-related deaths in the sixteenth century, 6.1 million in the seventeenth century, 7 million in the eighteenth, 19.4 million in the nineteenth, and 109.7 million in that most bloody of centuries—the twentieth.[59] The World Health Organization estimates that war-related injuries led to 310,000 deaths in 2000,[60] a year that does not stand out in our minds as being particularly bloody.

Nor does the suffering end there. Consider the number of people who are raped, assaulted, maimed, or murdered (by private citizens, rather than governments). About 40 million children are maltreated each year.[61] More than 100 million currently living women and girls have been subjected to genital cutting.[62] Then there is enslavement, unjust incarceration, shunning, betrayal, humiliation, and intimidation, not to mention oppression in its myriad forms.

For hundreds of thousands, the suffering is so great—or the acknowledgement of it so clear—that they take their own lives.

---

[57] Rummel, R. J., *Death by Government*, 69. His low estimate is 89 million, but the number could be as high as 260 million.

[58] Ibid. 9.

[59] Krug, Etienne G., Dahlbeg, Linda L., Mercy, James A., Zwi, Anthony B., and Lozano, Rafael., (eds.) *World Report on Violence and Health* (Geneva: WHO, 2002) 218.

[60] Ibid. 217.

[61] *The World Health Report 2002*, 80

[62] Toubia, Nahid, 'Female Circumcision as a Public Health Issue', *New England Journal of Medicine*, 331/11 (1994) 712.

For instance, 815,000 people are thought to have committed suicide in 2000.[63]

Pollyannaism leads most people to think that they and their (potential) children will be spared all this. And indeed there are some, although extremely few, who are lucky enough to avoid non-*inevitable* suffering. But everybody must experience at least some or other of the harms in the above catalogue of misery.

Even if there are some lives that are spared most of this suffering, and those lives are better than I have said they are, those (relatively) high-quality lives are exceedingly uncommon. A charmed life is so rare that for every one such life there are millions of wretched lives. Some know that their baby will be among the unfortunate. Nobody knows, however, that their baby will be one of the allegedly lucky few. Great suffering could await any person that is brought into existence. Even the most privileged people could give birth to a child that will suffer unbearably, be raped, assaulted, or be murdered brutally. The optimist surely bears the burden of justifying this procreational Russian roulette. Given that there are no real advantages over never existing for those who are brought into existence, it is hard to see how the significant risk of serious harm could be justified. If we count not only the unusually severe harms that anybody could endure, but also the quite routine ones of ordinary human life, then we find that matters are still worse for cheery procreators. It shows that they play Russian roulette with a *fully* loaded gun—aimed, of course, not at their own heads, but at those of their future offspring.

[63] Krug, Etienne, et al, *World Report on Violence and Health*, 185.

4

Having Children:
The Anti-Natal View

Philosophers. . .ought much rather to employ themselves in
rendering a few individuals happy, than in inciting the suffering species to multiply itself.

Martin in Voltaire's *Candide*[1]

The idea of bringing someone into this world fills me with
horror. . .May my flesh perish utterly! May I never transmit
to anyone the boredom and ignominies of existence!

Gustave Flaubert[2]

PROCREATION

I have argued so far that coming into existence is always a harm,
and that it is a serious harm. There is more than one way to
reach this conclusion. Those who reject the arguments in Chapter 2
that coming into existence is always a harm may nonetheless be

[1] Voltaire, *Candide*, (London: Penguin Books, 1997) 134–5.
[2] Flaubert, Gustave, Letter to Louise Colet, 11 December 1852, in *The Letters of Gustave Flaubert 1830–1857*, trans. Francis Steegmuller (London: Faber & Faber, 1979) 174.

persuaded by the arguments in Chapter 3 that our lives are actually very bad. Even those who deny that *all* lives are very bad should conclude from Chapter 3 that at least the overwhelming majority of lives are very bad. These conclusions must certainly have bearing on the question of having children (by which I mean the generation of children rather than rearing them).

No duty to procreate

Some people believe that there is a duty to procreate. There are various ways of understanding the (1) scope of, and (2) justification for this purported duty:

(1) Scope: A duty to procreate can be understood as (a) a duty to have *some* children, or it can be understood as (b) a duty to have *as many* children as one can.

(2) Justification: Purported duties to procreate could be based on (a) the interests of those brought into existence, or (b) other considerations, such as the interests of others, utility, divine commands, and so on.[3]

My arguments most powerfully challenge the duty when it is based on the interests of those brought into existence. If coming into existence is always a serious harm, then there can be no duty, based on the interests of potential people, to bring some and, a fortiori, as many as possible, of these people into existence. For a duty to procreate that is justified in this way to have any plausibility it must be limited to exclude cases where the only (additional) children one could have would lead lives that are so bad that they are not worth starting. That is to say, nobody could plausibly suggest that one had a duty, based on the interests of potential people, to bring some (and a fortiori as many as possible) of them into existence if their lives were not worth starting.

[3] For other grounds, see Smilansky, Saul, 'Is There a Moral Obligation to Have Children?', *Journal of Applied Philosophy*, 12/1 (1995) 41–53.

Since my arguments show that no lives are worth starting, the limitation excludes all lives from the scope of a duty to procreate. My arguments show, then, either that there is no duty to procreate or if there is such a duty that it is a purely theoretical duty that never applies in the real world. Even those who think that there are a few lives that were worth starting would have to abandon a duty to procreate. This is because both (a) one cannot tell in advance whether a life one starts will turn out to be one that was worth starting; and (b) the costs of error are so great, given how bad all other lives are.

My arguments pose a more indirect, but nonetheless substantial, challenge to a duty to procreate that is based on considerations other than the interests of those brought into existence. My arguments do not logically preclude these duties (and their having application in the real world). This is because one could acknowledge that coming into existence is a harm, even a serious one, and yet say that the considerations that ground the duty—such as the interests of others or divine commands—outweigh the harm. One *could* say this, but it is highly implausible if the harm of coming into existence is as severe as I have suggested. And it is more implausible the more harm one inflicts. This is why (1b) above based on (2b) is even more implausible than (1a) based on (2b): A duty to have as many children as one can, based on considerations other than the interests of those who are brought into existence, is even more implausible than is a duty to have some children, that is based on considerations other than the interests of those who are brought into existence.

Is there a duty not to procreate?

Do my arguments also show that it is actually wrong to have children? That is to say, is there a duty *not* to procreate, or is procreation neither obligatory nor prohibited? Many people will agree that there is *sometimes* a duty not to procreate—namely, in those cases where the child one brings into existence will have an unusually bad life. My question, however, is whether the duty not to bring people into existence applies to all possible people.

An affirmative answer would be sharply antagonistic to some of the most deeply seated and powerful human drives—the reproductive ones. In evaluating whether it is wrong to have children we must be acutely aware and suspicious of the power these drives have to bias us in their favour. At the same time, to embrace the view that procreation is wrong without due consideration of procreative interests would be rash.

At the outset, we must distinguish procreative interests from coital interests and parenting interests. Procreative interests are interests in bringing new people, one's genetic offspring, into existence.[4] Non-procreation comes at the cost of frustrating procreative interests. Not all people have such interests, but a great many people do.

Coital interests are interests in a kind of sexual union—coitus. The satisfaction of coital interests accounts for much procreation. Indeed many people are brought into existence not because their parents sought to satisfy their own procreative interests, but because their parents were satisfying their own coital interests. In other words, for a great number of people, their coming into existence is not so much the result of a parental decision to procreate, as a mere consequence of parental coitus. However, because coitus is possible without bringing anybody into existence (as happens, for example, when successful contraception is used), non-procreation need not come at the cost of frustrating coital interests (and a fortiori non-coital sexual interests). All it requires is some (contraceptive) care by one or both of the parties, and then only during the female's pre-menopausal life. The additional

---

[4] The phrase 'genetic offspring' is necessary because, for example, a fertility doctor's procreative interests are not fulfilled when he assists others in reproducing. (The phrase 'genetic offspring' is not restricted to those beings formed from one's own gametes, and can also include one's clone.)

effort that that care takes cannot begin to outweigh the harm of coming into existence, and thus we certainly cannot condone that baby-making that is a mere consequence (rather than a goal) of coitus.

Parenting interests are interests in rearing a child as well as interests in the relationship established with the (adult) children one has raised. Although these interests are usually fulfilled by rearing a child that is one's genetic offspring, one can rear children one has not produced oneself. Thus, the fulfilment of parenting interests does not always require the satisfaction of one's own procreative interests. At least while there are unwanted children, people can satisfy their interests in rearing children without producing any of their own. However, producing children of one's own is by far the easiest way of acquiring a child to rear. Adoption is an arduous process with considerable costs of an emotional and financial kind. Most of those who currently endure this process are those who cannot produce their own genetic child, although there are some people who elect to adopt in spite of their own fertility. For both fertile and infertile adopters, non-procreative rearing comes at the cost of the adoption process. If non-procreation became the norm (which it will not voluntarily become) and there were no unwanted children, then non-procreation would come at the cost of frustrating not only procreative interests but also parenting interests.

Children cannot be brought into existence for their own sakes. We do not need the argument in Chapter 2 to see why this is so, although that argument certainly shows that a person brought into existence cannot be the beneficiary of this instance of procreation. This is not to say that some procreators do not think that they are having children for those children's sakes. It is only to say that whatever such people might think, their having children cannot actually be for those children's sakes. If their reasons for having children are to bestow a benefit on those children, then they are mistaken.

People can have children for other reasons. Most people, where they even make a decision to have a child, make that decision, I suspect, in order to serve their own procreative and related interests. For some people, the decision may also, in part, be to serve the interests of others. These others may include one's own parents (who want to become grandparents), the tribe or the nation (that need new people in order to survive), or the state (that needs to be adequately peopled in order to function well). However, even in such cases, serving these other interests will usually coincide with serving the interests of the procreators themselves. Giving one's parents grandchildren silences the complaints about the absence of grandchildren. Making babies for the tribe, nation, or state earns one some status. But it is the procreative and related interests, I suspect, that account for most of the intentional baby-making. Parents satisfy biological desires to produce children and find fulfilment in nurturing and raising their children. When grown these children can become friends. They can provide grandchildren. And they are often an insurance policy for old age, caring for one in one's senility. Progeny provide parents with some form of immortality— through the genetic material, values, and ideas that parents pass on to their children, and which survive in their children and grand-children after the parents themselves are dead. Some of these are good reasons for people to want to have children, but none of them show why having children is not wrong. To the extent that these goods could be obtained without producing children of one's own, they cannot be used to defend baby-making. But at least some of these goods—most obviously the procreational interests—cannot be secured without making babies. Now the fact that procreation serves one's own interests is not enough to show that it is wrong. Serving one's own interests is not always bad. However, where doing so inflicts significant harm on others, it is usually not justified.

One way, then, to defend the having of children, even if one accepts my view that coming into existence is always a harm, would be to deny that that harm is great—that is, to deny the conclusion of Chapter 3. One could then argue that the harm is outweighed by the benefits to the parents and others. But what if one agrees that coming into existence is a *great* harm? Is there anything then that could be said to defend baby-making?

In defence of the permissibility of having children, it might be suggested that it is morally significant that most people whose lives go relatively well do not see their having come into existence as a harm. They do not regret having come into existence. My arguments suggest that these views may be less than rational, but that, it might be suggested, does not rob them of all their moral significance. Because most people who live (relatively) comfortable lives are happy to have come into existence, prospective parents of such people are justified in assuming that if they have children they too will feel this way. Given that it is not possible to obtain consent from people prior to their existence to bring them into existence, this presumption might play a key role in a justification for having children. Where we can presume that those whom we bring into existence will not mind that we do, we are entitled, the argument might go, to give expression to our procreational and other interests. Where these interests can be met by having either a child with a relatively good life or a child with a relatively bad life it would be wrong if the parents brought the latter into existence, even where that child would also not regret its existence. This is because if the prospective parents are to satisfy their procreational interests they must do so with as little cost as possible. The less bad the life they bring into being, the less the cost. Some costs (such as where the offspring would lead a sub-minimally decent life) are so great that they would always override the parents' interests.

Those cases in which the offspring turn out to regret their existence are exceedingly tragic, but where parents cannot reasonably foresee this, we cannot say, the argument would suggest, that they do wrong to follow their important interests in having children.

Things would be quite different, according to this argument, if the majority or even a sizeable minority of people regretted coming into existence. Under such circumstances the above justification for having children certainly would be doomed. However, given that most people do *not* regret their having come into existence, does the argument work? In fact, the argument is problematic (and not only for the reasons that Seana Shiffrin raises and which I mentioned in Chapter 2). Its form has been widely criticized in other contexts, because of its inability to rule out those harmful interferences in people's lives (such as indoctrination) that effect a subsequent endorsement of the interference. Coming to endorse the views one is indoctrinated to hold is one form of adaptive preference—where an interference comes to be endorsed. However, there are other kinds of adaptive preference of which we are also suspicious. Desired goods that prove unattainable can cease to be desired ('sour grapes'). The reverse is also true. It is not uncommon for people to find themselves in unfortunate circumstances (being forced to feed on lemons) and adapt their preferences to suit their predicament[5] ('sweet lemons'). If coming into existence is as great a harm as I have suggested, and if that is a heavy psychological burden to bear, then it is quite possible that we could be engaged in a mass self-deception about how wonderful things are for us. If that is so, then it might not matter, contrary to what is claimed by the procreative argument just sketched, that most people do not regret their having come into existence. Armed with a strong argument for the harmfulness of slavery, we would not take slaves' endorsement of their enslavement as a justification for their enslavement, particularly if we could point to some rationally questionable psychological phenomenon that explained the slaves' contentment.[6] If that is so, and if coming into existence is as great a harm as I have argued it is, then

---

[5] Often, although not always, this will start out as a way to save face, but even then it eventually can be internalized.

[6] There is just such a phenomenon in the case of kidnap victims, who often come to identify with their kidnappers.

we should not take the widespread contentment with having come into existence as a justification for having children.

To this it might be objected that a duty not to procreate is too demanding a requirement. I do not deny that forgoing procreation is a burden—that it is a lot to require of people, given their nature. But is it too much to require? I said earlier that many people would agree that there is sometimes a duty not to procreate—namely in those cases where the offspring would suffer terribly. In such cases many people are prepared to admit that it would be wrong to have a child. But notice that the burden for those who must desist from producing progeny in such cases is no lighter than the burden any other potential human breeder faces in forgoing having children. If the burden is not too great for the former, then it ought not to be too great for the latter. Where the difference is thought to lie is in the quality of life of the offspring. In other words, it is thought that non-procreation is required of those whose children's quality of life would be unacceptably low, but we cannot make such a demand of those whose offspring would be 'normal'. Notice, however, that this is not an argument about the magnitude of the burden of non-procreation, but rather one about when that burden may be imposed. I could accept that non-procreation should only be required when the children produced would lead very poor quality lives. This is because I have argued that *all* lives fall into this category. Those who think that a *few* lives do not fall into this category are not (much) better equipped to defend the objection that non-procreation is too demanding. This is because they must surely be moved by the fact that we cannot tell, when we deliberate about whether to bring somebody into existence, whether that life will be one of the few lives that is not of a very poor quality. It seems, then, that those who accept that coming into existence is a great harm and that there is a duty not to procreate in cases where the offspring would suffer great harm by being brought into existence must accept that a duty not to procreate is not too demanding.

If I am mistaken about this, however, and it is not immoral to have children, my arguments in Chapters 2 and 3 show, at the very least, that it is preferable not to have children. Although our potential offspring may not regret coming into existence, they certainly would not regret not coming into existence. Since it is actually very much not in their interests to come into being, the morally desirable course of action is to ensure that they do not.

PROCREATIVE FREEDOM

If it is merely preferable not to procreate, then there could still be a right to procreate. That is to say, one could be entitled—have a right—to do that which is sub-optimal.[7] However, if there is a duty not to procreate, then it seems that there can be no right to procreate. One cannot be entitled to do that which one has a duty not to do. Thus the argument that there is a duty not to produce children appears to threaten a commonly ascribed right to procreative freedom.[8] Is this really so?

Understanding the purported right

I shall understand a right to procreative freedom to be a right to choose whether or not to produce children. One aspect of this right—namely, the right not to produce children—clearly does not conflict with a duty not to procreate. If the right to procreative

---

[7] Maximizers, who collapse the distinctions between 'permissible', 'required', and 'supererogatory', would deny that we are ever entitled to do that which is sub-optimal. Thus, when I say that one could be entitled to do that which is sub-optimal I mean that one could do so by rejecting a maximizing view.

[8] Article 16 of the United Nations Universal Declaration of Human Rights (1948) says that 'men and women of full age. . .have the right to marry and found a family.' A right to 'found a family' is also ascribed by the International Covenant on Civil and Political Rights (Article 23) and the European Convention on Human Rights (Article 12). Taken literally, the right to 'found a family' is not unambiguously a right to procreate, for it is also possible to found a family by adoption, but it is clearly intended and understood that the right includes the procreative founding of a family.

freedom were understood to include only this aspect, then the right as a whole would not conflict with a duty not to have children. The conflict only arises when the right is both a right to make and a right not to make babies.

Moreover, I shall understand a right to procreative freedom to be a negative right—that is, a right not to be prevented from reproducing (with a willing partner) or not reproducing. In other words, I shall not understand it as a positive right to be assisted in having children or in avoiding having children. The question of assisted reproduction will be considered later in this chapter.

The conflict between a duty not to procreate and a purported right to procreate is starkest, and unavoidable, where the right in question is a moral right (assuming, as I do, that the duty not to procreate is a moral duty). If having children is morally wrong and there is therefore a moral duty not to have children, then there can be no moral right to have children. However, this leaves open the question whether there should be a legal right to have children. Having children may be morally wrong, but it may still be the case that there ought to be a legal right to do this wrong. One of the distinctive features of a legal right is that it allows somebody the liberty to do what may be, or regarded to be, wrong. A legal right to freedom of speech, for example, exists not to protect speech that everybody takes to be good and wise, but rather to protect speech that at least some take to be evil or stupid. One can think that somebody ought to have a legal right to say and do things that one personally regards as wrong. This fact, however, is insufficient by itself to show that there should be a legal right to procreative freedom. This is because there are many wrongs that there ought not to be a right to perform. For example, there ought not to be a legal right to murder, steal, or assault. The question, then, is whether or not bringing people into existence is the sort of wrong that should be legally protected. It is to that question that I now turn.

Grounding the right on autonomy

Clearly a right to produce children cannot be derived from a right *not* to produce children. One could have a right not to produce children without having a right *to* produce children. A purported right to procreate might, however, be based partially on considerations that also ground a right not to procreate. For instance, one might argue that an interest in one's autonomy might establish a presumption against interference with procreative choices. This argument can be bolstered by noting how important procreative decisions are for so many people. Procreative liberty tends to be highly valued, either in itself or as a means to parenting. Whether or not one reproduces can have a profound impact on the character and quality of one's life (although, pregnancy aside, it need not if one gives up for adoption children one produces, or if one adopts children one has not produced). It can affect one's sense of self. (For example, some people feel inadequate if they are unable to produce children of their genetic own.) Producing children can give meaning to some people's lives or have religious significance for them.

It is widely thought that these considerations are sufficient to justify a legal right to have children. However, those who think that there ought to be a legal right to have children but also accept the conclusion that it is always a harm to come into existence face the following difficulty. A legal right to have children is not an absolute entitlement but instead a very strong presumption in favour of having children. It is in the nature of a presumption that it can be defeated. Thus one defender of a right to procreative freedom notes that 'those who would limit procreative choice have the burden of showing that the reproductive actions at issue would create such substantial harm that they could justifiably be limited.'[9]

---

[9] Robertson, John, *Children of Choice* (Princeton: Princeton University Press, 1994) 24.

This is not very controversial. However, if one thinks that coming into existence is always a great harm, then the presumption in favour of a right to procreate is always defeated. But a right that is always defeated is not really a right. Although it might still be argued that it is a right in principle—a presumption that has to be defeated, even though it always is defeated—such rights are not suitably enshrined in law. To make the case that people ought to have a legal right to have children, one must surely demonstrate that there should be a presumption in practice, and not merely in principle, to choose whether to have children. The problem, then, is that a defeasible legal right to have children is not a plausible candidate for a legal right if the defeasibility conditions are always met.

Grounding the right on futility

One way in which a legal right to reproductive freedom might be defended without denying that coming into existence is always a harm would be to argue as follows. If a right to reproductive freedom were withheld in order to prevent harm to those who would be brought into existence, the state could then either simply let people exercise reproductive choices without having a right to do so, or it could actively prohibit reproduction. The first option would be pointless. If the point of withholding an entitlement to have children is to prevent the harm of bringing people into existence, why withhold an entitlement to have children only then to permit people to have children? Withholding the right would have to be linked, therefore, to a prohibition on having children.[10] However the argument in defence of a legal right to

---

[10] It is not lost on me that this will never be seriously considered by any state, at least with regard to all people within its borders. (There have clearly been states that have sought to restrict, prevent or prohibit the reproduction of undesired subsets of the population—blacks, Jews, 'imbeciles', and the lower classes, for example.) That no state would ever ask whether it should prohibit procreation by everybody

reproductive freedom might go, procreative prohibition simply would not work. People would find ways of breaking the law. To enforce the law, even partially and unevenly, the state would have to engage in highly intrusive policing and the invasions of privacy that that would entail. On the plausible assumption that coitus itself should not and cannot effectively be prohibited, the state would have to be able to distinguish between those, on the one hand, who conceived wittingly or negligently, and those, on the other hand, who conceived accidentally. In either case, the state would then have to require abortions. In the case of the unwilling, this would require physically restraining people and performing unwanted abortions on them. The threat of this would very likely drive pregnancy underground, with women gestating and giving birth on the quiet. This, in turn, would very likely increase pregnancy- and parturition-related morbidity and mortality. These sorts of moral costs are immense and there is a powerful case to be made for the view that they are not outweighed by the benefits. This is particularly so given that the full benefits are unlikely to be obtained, given that much procreation would not be prevented by a prohibition on producing children. The case would be strongest on a non-maximizing non-consequentialist view—the sort of view most friendly to rights—but it may also be true of maximizing consequentialist views, depending on just how much benefit and harm would be produced under each scenario.

Grounding the right on disagreement

In our world this argument seems sufficient to justify a legal right to procreative freedom and its constituent legal right to produce children. However, there is one further objection that needs to be

does not mean, however, that it is not a question worth asking. There may be all kinds of psychological, sociological, and political explanations for why procreation will never be universally prohibited in a state. It does not follow that this position is philosophically sound.

considered and met. We can certainly imagine a society in which non-procreation could be widely (even if not universally) ensured without the invasions of privacy and bodily intrusions described above. This would be so if a safe, highly effective contraceptive substance could be widely administered without the knowledge of the population or the consent of individual people—in the drinking water, for example, or by aerial spray. A state in which this were done would avoid the horrendous image of Orwellian surveillance, or forced sterilizations and abortions, and so on. Of course, it would still be violating personal autonomy, but this, we have already seen, is not sufficient to make the case for a legal right to produce children.

Can anything be said in defence of a right to reproductive freedom in a society in which procreation could be prevented in such unobtrusive and gentle ways? The strongest argument of which I can think, although not one without serious difficulties, is as follows. The view that coming into existence is always a harm is highly contested. Even if this view is nonetheless correct, the mere fact that it enjoys so little support shows that ordinary people can disagree about this. And where such disagreement exists about whether some action is (unjustifiably) harmful, the state should grant people the right to choose whether or not to engage in such actions. This argument suggests a qualification of the famous harm principle. According to this principle, in its unqualified form, states may prohibit activities only when they harm non-consenting parties. The qualification states that cases in which there is disagreement between ordinary people about whether some action is harmful do not fall within the scope of the principle.

There are some cases that seem to lend support to this view. Some might think that abortion is one such case. Pro-lifers, it might be said, believe that abortion unjustifiably harms the fetus and therefore should be prohibited under the harm principle. Some, but not all, pro-choicers might note that it is highly contested whether fetuses are morally considerable. Given this, they might argue, there ought to be a legal right to have an abortion even if it is the case that abortion is morally wrong.

However, there are other cases that call into serious question the proposed qualification to the harm principle. Consider the case of slavery in a slave-owning society—or at least that sort of slave-owning society where slavery is defended by a view that slaves are naturally suited to being slaves. In such a society we find large numbers of people who believe that slavery does not harm slaves. Indeed they might even believe that slavery benefits slaves. They might listen to the arguments of a few abolitionists that slavery is harmful to slaves, and reply that their claims are highly contested and thus exempted from the harm principle. Although that conclusion would be accepted readily by slavery's defenders, it is quite clear that neither the abolitionists in that society nor we who have the benefit of some temporal or geographic distance from slavery would be impressed by this argument. Surely there ought not to be a legal right to own slaves even when slavery's harmfulness is contested? This shows that the mere fact that an activity's status as harmful is contested does not show that the harm principle is inapplicable or that people should have a legal right to engage in it.

Grounding the right on reasonable disagreement

If the argument qualifying the application of the harm principle is to succeed, it must draw a distinction between whether an activity's status as harmful is *reasonably* contested and whether it is contested *simpliciter*. The mere fact of disagreement, even between ordinary people, is now not enough to restrict the harm principle. It must be shown that the disagreement is reasonable. But what is the mark of a reasonable disagreement? It cannot be reduced to the numbers of people holding differing views, for we have already seen how wrong even a majority of people can be in determining whether some action is sufficiently harmful to withhold a right to engage in it. Reasonable disagreement is thus not disagreement between ordinary people—people on the famous 'Clapham omnibus'. For a disagreement to be reasonable the reasons for one view on a matter must not be sufficiently stronger than reasons for conflicting views that accepting one of the conflicting views is actually (rather than merely perceived to be) unreasonable. Now the problem with this standard is that of differentiating between disagreements that are actually unreasonable and those that are only perceived to be so.

To see why this is so, consider the following. I think that there can be no reasonable disagreement about the harmfulness of chattel slavery, but many people in societies where such slavery is and was practised do not agree. I should like to think that their proximity to slavery clouds or clouded their judgement about its harmfulness, and that my perception is thus less distorted. Of course, proximity to a social norm does not always blind people. There were and are abolitionists in slave-owning societies. And many (but not enough) of us who were born and grew up in Apartheid South Africa but were not its direct victims did not think that there could be reasonable disagreement about the wrong of apartheid's racism. We saw our opponents, the defenders of apartheid, as manifestly unreasonable, blinded though they were to this. Consider, next, a currently more controversial case. I do not think that there can be reasonable disagreement that the cruel treatment inflicted on the billions of animals that are reared and killed for human consumption is wrong. I have carefully considered the philosophical arguments to the contrary and they have all the attributes of earlier desperate defences of racism. Clearly, however, those philosophers and others who defend the eating of meat do not agree with me. We have different perceptions about whether the disagreement is reasonable. How do we determine whether it is actually reasonable?

The foregoing is not to say that I take all those who disagree with me about anything to be unreasonable. Most pertinently, I cannot say, notwithstanding all my arguments, that those who deny that coming into existence is always a serious harm are unreasonable. I do think that they are wrong. However, until my position has been adequately tested against the very best objections one cannot assess whether my claim is one about which reasonable people can disagree or one with which it is unreasonable to disagree (or, for that matter, to agree!).

I have shown that a legal right to reproductive freedom is well justified in our actual world where the alternative involves appalling state invasions of privacy and bodily intrusions. My liberal instincts are troubled by the case of a society where all (or almost all) procreation could be prevented without such costs by involuntary and imperceptible contraception.[11] In such a case, the best defence of a right to reproductive freedom is the claim that there can be reasonable disagreement about whether coming into existence is a serious harm. If it turns out that there cannot be reasonable disagreement with the view that coming into existence is always seriously harmful, a legal right to procreative freedom would have to be questioned further. Those suspicious of state interference with personal freedom will be perturbed by this. The only solace in this case is that it is highly unlikely that liberal governments will rush into banning all procreation without more than overwhelming evidence in favour of such a ban. Governments will be so heavily disincentivized to prohibit all procreation,[12] unlike many other restrictions of an individual's freedom, that it is highly unlikely that a generalized prohibition will ever be implemented. It is even less likely that governments will rush prematurely into such a prohibition. It is much more likely that they will retain a right to procreate long after the

---

[11] I also have strong instincts that allowing people to cause suffering is wrong. These instincts pull in the opposite direction.

[12] As I mentioned in note 10 above, this generalized prohibition on procreation is to be distinguished from a prohibition on the procreation of undesired groups. But the latter kind of prohibition can be ruled out on other grounds, such as equality.

reasonableness of such a position has vanished (if it does indeed vanish). That delay in abandoning a legal right to procreate may be regrettable, but may be less regrettable than the alternative of prematurely abandoning such a right.

There is then, for now, a strong case for recognizing a legal right to reproductive freedom. I can envisage circumstances in which this case would crumble, but on account of the strong biases toward rejecting the view that coming into existence is a harm, the case would be in utter ruins before a rights-respecting state withdrew a legal right to reproduce. If matters were that clear, the loss of such a right would not be regrettable. Indeed, the loss of such a right in liberal societies will cease to be regrettable long before it ever is lost—if it is ever lost in a society that remains liberal. In the interim, we can defend a legal right to produce children even while thinking that there is a moral duty not to bring new people into existence.

That a legal right to reproductive freedom can be defended, at least for the moment, does not entail that it must retain its current parameters and weight. It is curious just how extensive and strong this right currently is in many jurisdictions. Causing or risking harm is often countenanced in the reproductive context to an extent that it would not be tolerated in any other context. Consider, for example, somebody who is either a carrier of or a sufferer from a serious genetic disease (such as Tay-Sachs or Huntington's) or an infectious disease (such as AIDS). Under at least some circumstances (or, for Huntington's, in all circumstances), this person's offspring stand a very high chance of being affected—twenty-five or fifty per cent in the case of genetic disorders and somewhere in between for infectious diseases such as AIDS. Whereas many societies ordinarily would not tolerate behaviour that put others at such risk of so serious a harm, there is often considerable tolerance of reproductive conduct that poses this kind of risk and harm.

Sometimes, as I indicated earlier, there is good reason for this. This is true, for example, when we cannot determine a person's culpability, at least without troubling invasions of privacy. Did he know that he was a carrier of the genetic disorder? Did she know that she was HIV positive? Did they employ reasonable contraceptive measures? These sorts of uncertainties often make it difficult to attach blame, let alone criminal sanctions, to irresponsible reproductive conduct. Unless one is willing to apply strict liability there would be similar problems with civil action. However, the tolerance for and even defence of risky and harmful reproductive behaviour extends further than this. It is thought to be wrong to prohibit, prevent, impede, or sometimes even discourage clearly culpable harmful reproduction even when we could do so without invasions of privacy.

Since there is no intrinsic reason why we should treat harm caused by reproduction any differently from comparable harm caused in other ways, we should be prepared to reconceive the limits of reproductive liberty. Given the bias in favour of reproductive freedom, it may help when considering whether any given risky reproductive practice should be protected by a right to reproductive freedom to ask ourselves whether we would think that taking that risk of that harm should be permitted in non-reproductive contexts. If we would not think that this should be permitted, then we should not judge it to be acceptable in reproductive contexts either.

No less a champion of liberty than John Stuart Mill argued that there should be some restrictions on the right to reproduce. He wrote about those people who produce children they cannot feed, but his arguments have more general application. He condemns the abundant number of 'writers and public speakers, including many of most ostentatious pretensions to high feeling, whose views of life are so truly brutish, that they see hardship in preventing paupers from breeding hereditary paupers in the workhouse itself'.[13] He argues that although the state may have

---

[13] Mill, John Stuart, *Principles of Political Economy* (London: Longmans, Green & Co., 1904) 220.

a duty to feed the destitute, 'it cannot with impunity take the feeding upon itself, and leave the multiplying free.'[14] Therefore he says later that there is 'evident justification for converting the moral obligation against bringing children into the world who are a burden to the community, into a legal one'.[15]

These are tough words that will not sit well with those liberals who want to indulge people engaging in grossly irresponsible reproductive conduct. This concern is not devoid of all foundation. There is a danger that the selective prohibition will be applied to the disempowered, while the powerful fail to hold themselves to the same standards.[16] But there is a cost to *not* prohibiting the most harmful reproduction. This, obviously, is the harm to those who are born as a result. Thus, the more appropriate way of dealing with very risky or harmful reproductive conduct is to prohibit it, where it is reasonable to do so, but to control for possible biases in the deliberative process leading to such prohibition.

DISABILITY AND WRONGFUL LIFE

Although many people are reluctant to restrict the right to reproductive freedom, there is widespread agreement that it is *sometimes* morally wrong to have children. It is commonly (although not universally) thought to be wrong, knowingly or negligently to bring into existence people who will have serious impairments such as blindness, deafness, or paraplegia. Seriously disabled lives are often thought not to be worth starting. Some have gone so far

[14] Ibid.

[15] Ibid. 229.

[16] Some may think that John Stuart Mill is guilty of such class discrimination in seeking to curb the breeding of the poor. However, he advocated contraception also for the 'genteel' classes. He was arrested, as a youth, for distributing handbills offering contraceptive advice (to rich and poor), a stunningly avant-garde activity in the early nineteenth century. See Schwartz, Pedro, *The New Political Economy of J.S. Mill* (London: Weidenfeld & Nicolson, 1972) 28, 245–54.

as to suggest that those culpably brought into existence with such conditions should be able to sue for 'wrongful life'.[17]

The non-identity problem and the disability rights objection distinguished

At the beginning of Chapter 2 I considered one objection to the view that people whose existence is inseparable from their severe impairments can be harmed by being brought into existence. The substance of this objection is the 'non-identity' problem. This objection, which I argued could be overcome, is to be distinguished from another objection to which I now turn. The non-identity objection does not deny that life with severe impairments is bad. Indeed it assumes it is. The problem arises because although such a life is bad, it is purportedly not possible to say that it is worse than the alternative of never existing and thus it cannot be said to be harmful to start such a life. The objection that I shall now consider—a disability rights objection—is different. It questions the very assumption of the non-identity problem. The objection can take various forms. In its boldest form, it denies that impairments (or at least some of them) are bad at all. In its more modest form it denies that impairments are sufficiently bad as to make lives with such impairments not worth starting. It follows from this that various attempts to prevent people with impairments from coming into existence, including pre-conception genetic screening, not to mention abortion, are wrong. More specifically, such attempts are said to express negative judgements about people with disabilities and the value of their lives. I shall now explain this disability rights objection and show how my arguments lend surprising and unusual support to the objection on the way to undoing it.

In discussing the disability rights objection, I shall focus on impairments that are serious but not the most severe. The disability rights

---

[17] Depending on the circumstances, the respondent would be either the parents or the doctors who failed to notify the parents of the fetus's condition.

objection would be highly implausible for those conditions, such as Tay-Sachs or Lesch-Nyhan, which are so bad that it is quite clearly in the interests of the sufferer to cease existing. To say of such lives that they are worth starting or, worse still, that they are not bad at all, would be to strain credulity beyond all reasonable bounds. Nor shall I consider the mildest impairments, such as colour-blindness, which many people would agree are not too bad. Instead I shall focus on impairments such as an inability to see, hear, or walk. These are impairments that are often beheld with (sometimes muted) horror by those who do not have them. Of course, many of those who *do* have these impairments would also rather not have them.[18] However, if faced with a choice between never existing and existing with the impairment, most of those who have the impairment would rather exist with the impairment. And even more of those with one of these impairments would rather continue existing with the impairment than cease to exist. This preference stands in starkest contrast to those without the impairments who say that they would rather die than become impaired in these ways. The latter preference is curious given how rarely it survives the acquisition of the impairment. Most of those who say that they would rather die than have an impairment such as paraplegia and who then acquire the impairment change their minds about whether death is preferable. It should be clear, then, why the serious but not most severe disabilities are the site of most contention and are thus the appropriate place to focus.

The 'social construction of disability' argument

One widely misunderstood argument advanced by disability rights advocates is the argument that disability is 'socially constructed'—that is, it is social arrangements that disable people. Many

---

[18] Not all those with impairments have this view. Most notably, some in the deaf community prefer to be deaf in much the same way that a French speaker might prefer being a Francophone to being an Anglophone.

who hear this view dismiss it too quickly. They assume that it is obviously false. That somebody cannot see or hear or walk, they say, is not socially constructed, but is instead a fact quite independent of society. This response misunderstands the argument, which is not that social arrangements make people blind or deaf or unable to walk. Instead, the argument is that there is a distinction to be drawn between inabilities and disabilities.[19] A blind person is unable to see, a deaf person unable to hear, and a paraplegic unable to walk. These inabilities become disabilities only in certain social environments. Thus, where buildings are not wheelchair accessible, for example, those unable to walk are disabled with respect to accessing the building. However, where buildings are wheelchair accessible no such disability exists for paraplegics. Disability rights advocates may note that everybody has inabilities. No human beings have the ability to fly (unaided by machines), but this fact does not disable the wingless, because buildings are made accessible to the wingless by means of ground-floor entrances and stairs, ramps, or lifts. We do not think about this because winglessness is the human norm. If most people had wings, and a few did not, then those few would be disabled if no accommodations were made for them. Thus the reason why those with impairments are disabled, where they are indeed disabled, is not because they have some inability, but rather because society is constructed in a way that excludes people with that inability.

[19] Actually, the distinction is usually between impairments and disabilities. (See, for example, Buchanan, Allen, Brock, Dan, Daniels, Norman, and Wikler, Daniel, *From Chance to Choice* (New York: Cambridge University Press, 2000) 285. Here they draw on Boorse, Christopher, 'On the Distinction between Disease and Illness', *Philosophy and Public Affairs*, 5/1 (1975) 49–68.) Impairments are negative departures from normal species functioning. Although I shall sometimes refer to 'impairments', I shall very often use 'inabilities' instead, as this may be a somewhat more powerful way of presenting the disability rights view. Because everybody, as I shall show, has some inabilities whereas not everybody has impairments as just defined, the contrast between inabilities and disabilities is a contrast between a characteristic we all have and a characteristic only the disabled have.

Now the significance of this is that it is not that the blind are unable to see or the deaf unable to hear that makes them disabled and therefore makes their lives go worse. Instead it is the fact that society does not accommodate their particular inabilities. In other words, what makes the lives of the blind or deaf go worse is the discriminatory social environment in which they find themselves.

The 'expressivist' argument

This 'social construction of disability' argument lends support to another disability rights argument, one that has been dubbed the 'expressivist' argument.[20] According to the expressivist argument, attempts to prevent people with impairments from coming into existence are objectionable because they express an inappropriate and hurtful message. This is the message that lives that are inseparable from impairments are not worth starting and that there should be no more people whose existence is inseparable from such impairments. This message, it is said, perpetuates prejudices about the value of the lives of those who lack sight, hearing, or the use of their legs, for example. To see better why the social construction of disability argument lends support to the expressivist argument, consider racial discrimination. Although race is not a perfect analogy,[21] there is some similarity between racial discrimination and discrimination on the basis of inabilities. For example, blacks are often disabled by their skin colour, but this is not because of any inherent property of their skin colour. Instead it is the result of obstacles that particular societies present to blacks. It is widely recognized that the fitting response to this disability is the removal of the obstacles, rather than the suggestion that no more black babies should be born. To the extent that

[20] By Buchanan, Allen, et al, *From Chance to Choice*. These authors do not themselves accept the argument.

[21] Because race is not itself generally an impairment. (There are some cases where it is: pale skin, for example, makes one more susceptible to skin cancer.)

the disabilities of the impaired are socially constructed, the fitting response to these disabilities is the removal of obstacles rather than the suggestion that there should be no more people with such impairments.

Responding to the disability rights arguments

These arguments raise a formidable challenge to ordinary quality-of-life assessments and judgements about what lives are not worth starting. I shall not consider the various responses that have been offered, because these responses all assume that lives without impairments are lives worth starting. (Indeed, such lives have even been referred to as 'perfect' individuals[22] and I have argued that no actual lives come anywhere near this description.) Instead I shall show how my argument that coming into existence is always a serious harm bolsters the disability rights position against its usual opponents while showing that both it and the position it criticizes are wrong.

One strength of the 'social construction of disability' argument is that it highlights the fact that there are normal human inabilities that go unnoticed in most people's assessments of quality of life. Part of the explanation for this is the obvious fact that the unusual generally stands out more than the usual. In this particular case it is partly because society, unsurprisingly, tends to get constructed in a way that fits well with the usual range of abilities and inabilities. It is only if special attention is given to unusual inabilities that these are accommodated. But this does not exhaust the explanation. As we saw in Chapter 3, various features of our psychology, including Pollyannaism, adaptation to misfortune, and comparison of one's own life with the lives of others, all conspire to make us think that our lives are much better than they really are. We are blinded, then, to the negative features of our own lives. We can

[22] Buchanan, Allen, et al, *From Chance to Choice*, 272.

now see that this problem is worse, in some ways, for those with usual inabilities. Not only does the social structure not show up these inabilities but neither are there other people without these inabilities with whom they can compare themselves or who will compare themselves with them.[23]

Disability rights advocates are correct to note that usual inabilities are ignored in quality-of-life assessments. They are mistaken, however, in taking that response to normal inabilities as the standard and in wanting to ignore unusual inabilities too. Instead, as the discussion in Chapter 3 shows, we should be considering all inabilities in assessing the quality of lives. While it is true that the social environment does minimize the impact that usual inabilities have on quality of life, many of them do nonetheless adversely impact on quality of life. Paraplegics may require special access to public transport, but the inability of everybody to fly or to cover long distances at great speed means that even those who can use their legs require transportation aids. Our lives surely go less well for being so dependent. Our lives also go less well because we are susceptible to hunger and thirst (that is unable to go without food and water), heat and cold, and so on. In other words, even if disability is socially constructed, the inabilities and other unfortunate features that characterize normal human lives are enough to make our lives go very badly—indeed much worse than we usually recognize. Socially constructed disability makes some lives still worse and we should certainly join disability rights advocates in seeking reasonable accommodations that would minimize or remove such disability. That would not be enough, however, to make any lives worth starting.

[23] That those with the impairments nonetheless have favourable views of their quality of life could be explained in two ways. Either Pollyannaism and adaptation outweigh the unfavourable comparison with those free of the impairment, or those people with impairments focus on comparisons with those who are still worse off than they are (which itself would be an instance of Pollyannaism).

Disability rights advocates also correctly note that quality-of-life assessments differ quite markedly between those who have impairments and those who do not. Many of those without impairments tend to think that lives with impairments are not worth starting (and may even not be worth continuing) whereas many of those with impairments tend to think that lives with these impairments are worth starting (and certainly are worth continuing). There certainly does seem to be something self-serving about the dominant view. It conveniently sets the quality threshold for lives worth starting above that of the impaired but below normal human lives. But is there anything less self-serving about those with impairments setting the threshold just beneath the quality of *their* lives? Disability rights advocates argue that the threshold in most people's judgements about what constitutes a minimally decent quality of life is set too high. However, the phenomenon of discrepant judgements is equally compatible with the claim that the ordinary threshold is set too low (in order that at least some of us should pass it). The view that it is set too low is exactly the judgement that we can imagine would be made by an extra-terrestrial with a charmed life, devoid of any suffering or hardship. It would look with pity on our species and see the disappointment, anguish, grief, pain, and suffering that marks every human life, and judge our existence, as we (humans without unusual impairments) judge the existence of bedridden quadriplegics, to be worse than the alternative of non-existence. Our judgements of what constitutes acceptable limits of suffering are profoundly influenced by the psychological phenomena I described in Chapter 3. They are accordingly unreliable. However, it is not only the dominant judgement that is unreliable. The judgements of those with impairments are also unreliable. The arguments I advanced in Chapter 3 showed that all actual lives are much worse than we think, and that none of our lives are worth starting.

This conclusion has an interesting implication for the expressivist argument. It will be recalled that according to the expressivist argument attempts to avoid bringing people with impairments into existence expresses an offensive view that there should be no such people and that such lives are not worth starting. In a way my conclusion simply extends the scope of the 'offensive' message, applying it to all people. Thus I join the opponents of the expressivist argument in agreeing that lives with impairments are not worth starting, but I do so in a way that will not be pleasing to those opponents. That is because I deny that *any* lives are worth starting. Curiously, however, this may make my view less rather than more offensive to disability rights activists. Whether or not it has this effect will depend on whether the offence and hurt of the expressed message rest on the apparently self-serving, exclusionary, or bigoted judgement that 'we are okay and you are not'. If that is indeed the basis for the hurt, then my view, though saying that more lives are not worth starting, will be less offensive to those with impairments. This is because I am making the claim not only about their lives, but about everybody's life, including my own.

The message that there should be no more lives like one's own need not be as personally threatening as some people think. To understand why this is so, consider again, the distinction I drew in Chapter 2 between future-life cases and present-life cases. The judgements we make about future-life cases—judgements about whether lives are worth starting—are (and should be) made at a different level from judgements about present-life cases—judgements about whether lives are worth continuing. To say that another life qualitatively like one's own is not worth starting is not (necessarily) to say that one's own life is not worth continuing. Nor is it to undermine the value that one's life has to oneself. Of course, it is to say that it would have been better had one's own life not started, but that is only threatening if one contemplates one's never existing from the perspective of one's existing. Put another way, it is to consider a future-life decision about one's own life from a present-life perspective. But that is a mistake. It is to fail to consider truly the counterfactual case where one does not (yet) exist, and thus has no interest whatsoever in coming into existence.

Wrongful life

Considering only the arguments in Chapters 2 and 3, it might seem that *anybody*, not only those with unusually severe impairments, should be able to sue for wrongful life. However, I have argued earlier in the current chapter that (at least for now) there should be a (legal) right to procreative freedom. Although this right must be defeasible, it cannot be defeated routinely without the case for its very existence being undermined. If that is the case, then there should be a legal right to produce children that reasonably can be expected to have *relatively* good lives. If the argument for such a right is strong, then the case for allowing wrongful life suits by simply anybody is weakened. However, it is not entirely eliminated. It could still be argued that although people should be legally entitled to have children, they should not be immune from civil suit should those children be unhappy with having been brought into existence. However, this would be a difficult case to make. For a wrongful life case to be well founded there would have to be evidence that the respondent acted unreasonably, but that would be hard to show so long as the case for a legal right to have children had not crumbled. Remember that the appropriateness of such a right ultimately rests on the possibility of reasonable disagreement.

So much for wrongful life suits by people with relatively good lives. Should those with impairments be able to sue for wrongful life against those who culpably brought them into existence in such condition? The case for such suits rests on the plausible view that if one is going to have children, then one should rather have children whose lives will go better than children whose lives will go worse. But here we must be cautious. The disability rights arguments show that those without impairments tend to overestimate how bad life is with the impairments. Now obviously those who bring wrongful life suits on their own behalf do not think their quality of life is overestimated. However, wrongful life suits are often brought on behalf of those who are not competent to sue. There is a real danger in such cases that unimpaired[24] judges and juries will judge by their own unreliable standards. Even where somebody sues for his own wrongful life, it is likely that judges and juries will sympathize, because of their biases, with his view even where it diverges from others with such disabilities. Some may not see this as a problem because they might take a person's own assessment of his quality of life as being decisive. In this case, the views of other impaired people may be viewed as irrelevant. However, because a wrongful life case must demonstrate that the culpable party was unreasonable, the views of other people with such conditions are relevant. If wrongful life suits are to be allowed only in cases of unusual hardship, then assessment of what constitutes unusually poor quality of life cannot be idiosyncratic.

The disability rights arguments pose another problem for wrongful life suits. If lives with impairments are only a little worse than other lives, then they may not be bad enough to be distinguished from normal lives for the purposes of wrongful life suits. Indeed there may be some lives without bodily or psychological impediments that are worse than some lives with impairments. A life of extreme poverty, for example, may be worse than a life of a blind person who has access to reasonable resources. The life of a fulfilled, happy paraplegic may be of a higher quality than the life of an unfulfilled, unhappy able-bodied athlete.

Notwithstanding the above concerns, there may be some scope for wrongful life suits. To judge the strength of the case we would have to control for the sorts of errors just mentioned. We can imagine lives, however, of such immense suffering—suffering that

---

[24] That is, those who lack what are usually regarded as impairments.

should have been anticipated and would have been avoided but for maliciousness or negligence—where wrongful life suits are entirely apt.

ASSISTED AND ARTIFICIAL REPRODUCTION

I turn now from questions about disability and wrongful life to questions about assisted and artificial reproduction, on which my arguments in Chapters 2 and 3 also have some bearing.

The terms 'assisted reproduction' and 'artificial reproduction' are often used interchangeably, but they are not synonymous. Artificial reproduction refers to reproduction by non-coital means.[25] The idea here is that coitus is the natural way of bringing sperm and ovum together. If sperm and ovum are brought together via some other means, then it is artificial rather than natural. Thus artificial insemination is artificial because insemination is effected by means of an artefact rather than a (natural) body part. *In vitro* fertilization, followed by embryo transfer, is also artificial by this standard. So too is cloning, which does not involve a union of sperm and ovum at all, and is achieved by technological intervention.

Assisted reproduction, as the term suggests, refers to cases where those reproducing are assisted in their reproductive activity. Although most instances of artificial reproduction are also instances of assisted reproduction, whether all are depends on what one understands assistance to be. A couple that reproduces by artificial insemination need not be assisted at all, unless one takes the inseminating implement to be a relevant form of assistance. There are also possible cases of assisted reproduction that are not cases

[25] The one problematic case for this account is that of parthenogenesis, where an ovum spontaneously undergoes division. However, we can ignore such a case on the grounds that these cases do not come to term.

of artificial reproduction. Treatment for erectile dysfunction, for example, might be viewed as assisting people with reproduction (although it does have other purposes), yet would not fall within the scope of artificial reproduction as it is usually understood.

Reproductive ethics and sexual ethics

Some people judge artificial reproduction to be unethical because they think that the only acceptable way to conceive a child is via a sexual expression of mutual love within the confines of a marriage. It is not sufficient, on this view, that the reproducing parties are married to one another, love one another, and seek to reproduce as an expression of their love. The couple's mutual love, expressed sexually, must be the proximate cause of the child's conception. I cannot see how this last requirement could be defended adequately. What is so important about a sexual expression of love that is a necessary condition for the ethically acceptable production of a child?

So much for the view that reproduction must be sexual—what we might call the 'sexual view of reproductive ethics'. Many of those who accept this view, along with other people who do not, accept the opposite conditional: that sexual interactions must be procreative. We might call this the 'reproductive view of sexual ethics'. On this view, sex can *only* be acceptable morally if it is directed towards reproduction. This is not to say that all sexual acts that produce a child are morally acceptable. Rape and adultery, for example, can produce offspring but typically would not be morally acceptable. Reproductive possibility is a necessary but not a sufficient condition for sex to be acceptable. The reproductive view of sexual ethics does not claim that all coital acts that do not result in a child are wrong. Many sexual reproductive attempts simply fail. Instead the reproductive view of sexual ethics maintains that a sexual act must be of the reproductive sort. This requirement rules out non-coital sex, including oral and anal sex.

Curiously, and inexplicably, it is not thought to rule out coitus within a marriage in which one of the partners is infertile.

I mention this view because it has many adherents and because my arguments pose an unusual challenge to it. My arguments turn the reproductive view of sexual ethics on its head. Most of those who reject the reproductive view do so because they think that sex *need not* hold procreative possibility in order to be morally acceptable. My arguments produce a much stronger conclusion—for sex to be morally acceptable it *must not* be reproductive. In other words, sex can only be morally acceptable if it is not reproductive. We might call this the 'anti-reproductive view of sexual ethics'. To clarify, this view does not maintain that all non-reproductive sex is morally acceptable. Non-reproduction is a necessary but not sufficient condition. Nor does it claim that coitus is wrong, but only that those coital acts where procreation is not prevented are wrong. But what does it mean to say that procreation is 'not prevented'? It can refer to cases where no (or poor quality) contraception was used and which result in a new person being brought into existence. Does it also refer to cases where a reliable method of contraception was used, but which happened to fail in some instance? It certainly seems difficult to hold people responsible for merely possible, though extremely rare, outcomes of their actions. Is driving a car wrong because my brakes *could* fail and a pedestrian could die, or am I only responsible if I drive a car that I fail to keep well-serviced and of which I consequently lose control, killing a pedestrian?

The question about rare contraceptive failure would be more pressing if the harm of coming into existence were inflicted at the time of conception. However, as I shall argue in the next chapter (on abortion), this is the wrong way to date the harm of coming into existence. Contraceptive failure still leaves open abortive possibility. There are parts of the world, of course, where abortive possibilities are limited. In such cases the duty to prevent conception would be stronger, but where conception does occur despite such attempts those preventing abortion would bear moral liability for bringing a new person into existence.

To summarize the previous paragraphs, I reject both the sexual view of reproductive ethics and the reproductive view of sexual ethics. I do so in an unusual way—via an anti-reproductive view of both reproductive and sexual ethics—rather than by means of the usual response, which we might call the 'neutral view'. (See Tables 4.1 and 4.2.)

Table 4.1. Reproductive ethics

Sexual view	Neutral view	Anti-reproductive view
Reproduction can only be morally acceptable if it is sexual.	It makes no moral difference whether reproduction is sexual or not.	Reproduction is never morally acceptable.

Table 4.2. Sexual ethics

Reproductive view	Neutral view	Anti-reproductive view
Sex can only be morally acceptable if it is reproductive.	It makes no moral difference whether sex is reproductive or not.	Sex can be morally acceptable only if it is not reproductive.

If it is wrong to bring new people into existence then it makes no difference whether one brings them into existence sexually or otherwise. And if bringing new people into existence is wrong, then child-producing sex is wrong.

The tragedy of birth and the morals of gynaecology[26]

The scope of the anti-reproductive view of reproductive ethics extends not only to those who are reproducing, but also to

[26] This heading, a play on Friedrich Nietzsche's *The Birth of Tragedy and the Genealogy of Morals*, was suggested to me by Allen Buchanan.

anybody who might assist them in this. In other words, my arguments pose a challenge to infertility medicine and its practitioners. More specifically, my arguments suggest that it is wrong to help somebody inflict the harm of bringing somebody into existence.

It does not follow from this that providing fertility treatment should be illegal. If there should be a negative right to reproductive freedom, then state or other interference with a person's efforts to seek out fertility assistance or another person's willingness to provide such help, would be precluded. This does not mean that fertility specialists do no wrong in helping to bring new people into existence. It means only that they should have the legal freedom to do so. This freedom is derivative from their patients' negative rights to reproductive freedom.

However, a negative legal right not to be prevented from seeking assistance in reproduction does not ground a positive legal or moral right to such assistance. Nor, it seems, can such a right be justified in some other way if my arguments are sound. Thus people should not be able to demand, as a matter of right, that a medical practitioner with the relevant expertise provide assistance in bringing new people into existence. Nor may they demand of the state that it provide resources for such services or the underlying research. Indeed, the state should not provide such resources. Even where resources are not limited, the state should not be helping to harm. Where resources are limited, they should be devoted to preventing and alleviating harm rather than causing it.

TREATING FUTURE PEOPLE AS MERE MEANS

There have been a few cases in which people have had a child in order to save an existing child. For example, a couple may have a child who develops leukaemia. A bone marrow transplant is required and there are no suitable donors. The couple decides to produce a new child that could serve as a donor. Sometimes, the plan is a mere lottery. The parents conceive and bring to term a child that they merely hope will be a suitable match. Either way they will love and rear it. Sometimes, though, there is greater planning. Embryos are tested to determine whether the child that would result would be a suitable match and only implanted if they would be. Or fetuses are tested and aborted if they will not grow into a child that will be a suitable donor.

Each of these options is more controversial than the preceding one. There are some people who are troubled even by the first option—having a child that one hopes, but does not ensure, will be a suitable match. The objection is that the parents treat the future child as a mere means to the ends of the existing child and this is accordingly in violation of the Kantian requirement not to treat people merely as a means.

This same objection has been raised against reproductive cloning. It has been said that the clone is not brought into existence for his or her own sake but rather for the sake of others, including, very often, the being that is cloned. The clone is treated as a mere means to the ends of the being cloned. This, it is said, is unacceptable.

What those who raise the Kantian-like objection routinely ignore is that in so far as it applies to cloning and cases of having a child in order to save a child, it applies at least as much to ordinary cases of having children. This is true irrespective of whether one accepts that coming into existence is always a serious harm. Clones and those children who are produced to save the life of a sibling are not brought into existence for their own sakes. This, however, is no different from any children. Children are brought into existence not in acts of great altruism, designed to bring the benefit of life to some pitiful non-being suspended in the metaphysical void and thereby denied the joys of life.[27] In so far as children are ever

[27] Benatar, David, 'Cloning and Ethics', *QJMed*, 91 (1998) 165–6.

brought into existence for anybody's sake it is never for their own sake.

Thus cloning is, at least in this regard, no more problematic than ordinary reproduction. Now it might be suggested that cloning is sometimes worse because, where it is done for the sake of the person cloned, it is also an act of narcissism. The being cloned wants a physical replica of himself. Thus the clone is treated as a means to the *narcissistic* ends of the person cloned. Now there might indeed be some people who will wish to have themselves cloned for narcissistic reasons, but others may want to be cloned for other reasons (perhaps because it is their only or best chance of reproducing). Moreover, the argument from narcissism assumes that ordinary reproduction is not narcissistic. But why should we think that that is always the case? There could well be something self-adulating in the desire to produce offspring. Those who adopt children or do not have children at all could advance the narcissistic objection against non-clonal reproduction with as much (or as little) force as non-clonal reproducers do in criticizing cloning. They could argue that it is narcissistic for a couple to want to create a child in their combined image, from a mixture of their genes. The point is that both cloning and usual methods of reproduction may be narcissistic, but neither is it the case that each kind of reproduction must necessarily be characterized in this way.

Cloning, therefore, is no more problematic than regular reproduction in this regard. It is also no less problematic. By contrast, the case of having a child in order to save a child *is* less problematic than ordinary cases of reproduction. In ordinary reproduction people produce children (a) to satisfy their procreative or parenting interests; (b) to provide siblings to existing children; (c) to propagate the species, nation, tribe, or family; or (d) for no reason at all. These are all clearly weaker reasons for producing a child than is the goal of saving the life of an existing person. It certainly seems strange to think that it is acceptable to have a child for no reason at all, but wrong to have a child in order to save somebody's life. If the latter is a case of unjustifiably treating one person as a means to the ends of others, then this must apply even more forcefully to all other cases of having children.

5

Abortion:
The 'Pro-Death' View

Cursed be the day on which I was born: let not the day on which my mother bore me be blessed. Cursed be the man. . . because he slew me not from the womb; so that my mother might have been my grave and her womb always great. Why did I come out of the womb to see labour and sorrow?

Jeremiah 20:14–18.

And Job spoke, and said, 'Oh that the day had perished wherein I was born, and the night which said "There is a man child conceived." Let that day be darkness. . .As for the night, let darkness seize upon it. . .because it did not shut up the doors of my mother's womb. . .Why did I not die from the womb? Why did I not perish when I came out of the belly?. . .For now should I have lain still and been quiet. . .or as a hidden untimely birth I had not been; as infants that never saw light.'

Job 3: 2–4, 6, 10, 11, 13, 16.

I have argued that it is better never to come into existence, but I have said nothing so far about *when*—that is, at what stage in the human developmental process—one comes into existence. It is to this question (and related issues) that I now turn. Much rests on the answer to this question. Combining some common, highly plausible answers with the view that it is better never to come into existence generates quite radical implications for the abortion question.

As things stand, most people tend to think that some reason needs to be provided *for* having or performing an abortion. Defenders of abortion maintain that adequate reason, at least at the earlier stages of gestation, need be no more than a preference of the woman who has the abortion. Nevertheless, it remains true that here the preference defeats a presumption in favour of continuing the pregnancy. Some of those who procure or perform abortions take abortion to be regrettable even when justifiable.

The moral presumptions must be reversed if (1) coming into existence is a harm, *and* (2) somebody has not yet come into existence at the particular stage of gestation when the abortion is to be performed. If both of these conditions are met, then the burden of proof is shifted to those who would *not* abort (at the specified stage of gestation). The *failure* to abort is what must be defended. The greater the harm of existence, the harder it will be to defend that failure. If a third condition is met—(3) coming into existence (in ordinary cases) is as great a harm as I have suggested it is—then the failure to abort (at the specified gestational age) may never, or almost never, be justified.

I have already considered conditions (1) and (3) in earlier chapters. Thus I focus here only on condition (2). Those who adopt the conservative view that one comes into existence at conception will maintain that there is no stage during gestation at which somebody has not yet come into existence. In advancing an argument that one begins to come into existence only quite late in the gestational process, I shall reject the conservative view along with some other views.

Before defending the claim that one begins to come into existence at a relatively late stage in the gestational process, I must clarify what I mean by 'coming into existence'. This phrase has different senses—including what we might call the *biological* sense and the *morally relevant* sense. By the biological sense is meant the beginning of a new organism, and by the morally relevant sense is meant the beginning of an entity's morally relevant interests. It is the latter sense that I am employing. In doing so, I am not presupposing that there *must* be different times at which some entity, even a human being, comes into existence in these different senses. The two senses are simply two things one might *mean* by the phrase. Whether they *refer* to the same time or different times is a distinct matter—a matter to which I shall soon turn.

There is *something* to be said for the view that we come into existence in the biological sense at the time of conception. Prior to conception there is only a sperm and an ovum. As these are both necessary for bringing somebody into existence, but because they are distinct entities prior to conception, they cannot be identical with the being that will be brought into existence. Two cannot be identical with one. Thus we cannot speak of a new organism as having come into existence prior to conception. Put another way, each one of us was once a zygote, but none of us was ever a sperm or an (unfertilized) ovum.[1] Although one could not have come into existence (in the biological sense) *prior* to conception, there is some room for doubting that it is the time of conception *at* which a single new organism arises. This is because of the possibility of monozygotic twinning, which persists for about fourteen days after conception. One would have to date the beginning of a being's irreversible biological individuality still later if one wished to take the phenomenon of conjoined twins into account.[2]

However, the question when one comes into existence in the biological sense need not detain us. This question can be bypassed

[1] This is *part* of what creates the absurdity in those who, joking about their conception, say that they remember going to a picnic with their father and coming back with their mother.

[2] For more on this, see Singer, Peter, Kuhse, Helga, Buckle, Stephen, Dawson, Karen, and Kasimba, Pascal (eds.) *Embryo Experimentation* (Cambridge: Cambridge University Press, 1990) 57–9, 66–6.

if one is interested, as I am, in the morally relevant sense and if, as I shall argue, one comes into existence in the morally relevant sense after even the latest reasonable estimate of when one comes into existence in the biological sense.

To determine when one acquires morally relevant interests, which is necessary for determining when one comes into existence in the morally relevant sense, we need to examine different senses of 'interest'.

FOUR KINDS OF INTERESTS

Philosophers have offered varying interpretations of what interests are, and what sorts of entities can have them. I shall discern four incremental senses of 'interest', before showing how the taxonomies of others relate to mine. Then I shall consider which kinds of interests are morally relevant.

1. *Functional interests:* The first sort of interest is that which an artefact, such as a car or a computer, is sometimes said to have. Because artefacts have functions, some things can promote and others impede those functions. Those things that facilitate an artefact's functioning are said to be good for the artefact, or to be in its interests, and those things that compromise its functioning are said to be bad for it, or against its interests. Thus, rust is bad for a car and having wheels is good.

2. *Biotic interests:* Plants have a different kind of interest. Like artefacts, they function, and their functioning can be fostered or impaired. However, unlike artefacts, plants are alive. Their functions and associated interests are biotic.

3. *Conscious interest:* Conscious animals also function, and as with plants, their functions are biological. But there is something that it *feels* like to be a conscious being. The associated interests I shall call conscious interests. But this

term requires clarification. By conscious interest I do not mean an interest that one consciously has—that one is explicitly aware of having—but rather an interest that can only be had by those who are conscious. One may, for instance, have an interest in avoiding pain, without being aware that one has such an interest.

4. *Reflective interests:* Some animals—typically most humans— are not only conscious, but are also characterized by various higher-order cognitive capacities, including self-awareness, language, symbolization, and abstract reasoning. Such animals are not only conscious, but are also 'reflective'. They have interests in the reflective sense that they can be explicitly interested in their interests.

I have stated above that these four senses of interest are *incremental.* I can now explain what I meant by that. The interests have been listed in ascending order. The higher sorts of interests incorporate the lower ones. Thus, artefacts have 'mere' (functional) interests. Living things have biotic interests. Conscious beings have conscious biotic interests, and 'reflective' beings have self-conscious biotic interests.[3]

The taxonomy of interests employed by some philosophers effectively collapses some of the above distinctions. For instance, Raymond Frey, in arguing against (non-human) animals' having moral standing, has distinguished between (a) interest as well-being and (b) interest as want.[4] The word is used in the former sense when one says that 'X is in Y's interests', and in the latter

---

[3] As a counter-example, some might want to point to the prospect of conscious or even self-conscious artefacts—Artificial Intelligence. Although this case obviously requires considerable discussion, I suggest here that any artefact that were genuinely conscious would qualify in virtue of this as being alive in the relevant sense, even though it may be somebody's artefact rather than somebody's offspring. I have the same concerns about bringing conscious machines into existence as I do with bringing conscious humans or animals into existence.

[4] Frey, R. G., 'Rights, Interests, Desires and Beliefs', *American Philosophical Quarterly*, 16/3 (1979) 233–9.

sense when one says 'Y has an interest in X.' In Professor Frey's view, interests in the first sense can be attributed to artefacts, plants,[5] and animals, given that things can be good or bad for any of these entities. However, he says that (interests as) wants can be ascribed only to those beings, such as (adult and lingual child) humans, that are capable of language.[6] He argues as follows:

(1) To want or desire X, one must believe that one does not currently have X.

(2) To believe that one does not have X is to believe that 'I have X' is false.

(3) One cannot have such a belief unless one knows how language connects with the world.

(4) One cannot know how language connects with the world if one does not have language.

(5) Therefore, beings that do not have language cannot have desires.

Professor Frey's interest as well-being encompasses the first three senses of interest that I discerned. His interest as want and what I have called reflective interests would be borne by the same kinds of beings, even though these two senses of interest are not the same. That is, 'interest as want' and 'reflective interest' do not have the same meaning, but the same kinds of beings would bear them (on his view).

The environmental philosopher, Paul Taylor, also distinguishes between (a) X being in Y's interests and (b) Y having an interest in X,[7] but he departs from Raymond Frey in the kinds of entities to which he attributes interests in these different senses.[8] In doing so,

---

[5] He does not explicitly mention plants, but given his arguments we can confidently include them in this category.

[6] Given the incremental nature of the interests, beings with language obviously have the lesser interest as well-being (the (a)-sense) in addition to interest as want (the (b)-sense).

[7] Taylor, Paul W., *Respect for Nature* (Princeton: Princeton University Press, 1986) 63.

[8] Ibid. 60–71.

he collapses my taxonomy in a different way from Professor Frey. Professor Taylor claims that not only humans but also conscious animals can have interests in the (b)-sense. But, like humans and conscious animals, non-conscious animals and plants can have a good of their own. Things can be good or bad *for* them. They can have interests in the (a)-sense. The same, he says, is not true of mere things and artefacts. When we speak about what is good for a machine we must make reference not to the machine's own purposes but to the purposes invested in it by those who make or use it. On this view, mere things and artefacts have interests in no sense.

Whereas Paul Taylor denies interests (in every sense) only to mere things and artefacts, Joel Feinberg denies interests also to non-conscious biotic entities, such as plants.[9] He denies, in other words, that there can be interests in either the functional or biotic sense. This is because he denies that artefacts or plants really have a good (even though we do sometimes speak as though they do). Professor Feinberg does not employ, and therefore implicitly collapses, the distinction between interests in the (a)-sense and interests in the (b)-sense. It is on precisely these grounds that Tom Regan[10] takes issue with him. Professor Regan, who defends the distinction between interests in the (a)-sense and interests in the (b)-sense, refers to them, respectively, as Interests$_1$ and Interests$_2$. He argues that we cannot infer from the fact that artefacts and plants do not have a certain kind of good—a conscious good, or 'happiness'—that they do not have any kind of good at all. Like

[9] Feinberg, Joel, 'The Rights of Animals and Unborn Generations', *Rights, Justice and the Bounds of Liberty* (Princeton: Princeton University Press, 1980) 159–84. (This essay first appeared in William T. Blackstone (ed.) *Philosophy and Environmental Crisis* (Athens: University of Georgia Press, 1974) 43–68.) Following Professor Feinberg, Bonnie Steinbock takes the same view. See her *Life Before Birth* (New York: Oxford University Press, 1992) 14–24.

[10] Regan, Tom, 'Feinberg on What Sorts of Beings Can Have Rights?', *Southern Journal of Philosophy*, 14 (1976) 485–98. Robert Elliot offers a defence of Joel Feinberg in his 'Regan on the Sorts of Beings that Can Have Rights', *Southern Journal of Philosophy*, 16 (1978) 701–5.

Raymond Frey, Tom Regan thinks that artefacts, plants, animals, and humans can all have interests in some or other sense (although these two philosophers disagree about which kinds of interests are morally relevant).

The relationship between the above taxonomies can be represented more clearly in diagrammatic form, as shown in Figure 5.1.

(a) X is in Y's interests (Interests$_1$)	(b) Y has an interest in X (Interests$_2$)	
Artefacts Plants Animals	Humans	Raymond Frey
Plants	(Conscious) Animals Humans	Paul Taylor
(Conscious) Animals Humans		Joel Feinberg
Artefacts Plants	(Conscious) Animals Humans	Tom Regan

Figure 5.1.

It is a mistake to attempt to settle the question whether some kind of entity is morally considerable *merely* by determining *whether* it has interests. Having interests may be necessary for having moral standing, but it is not sufficient. If an entity does not have interests then it cannot be harmed or benefited and thus it cannot have moral standing. However, it is logically possible for an entity to have interests, but only morally irrelevant ones. The crucial question, then, is which kinds of interests are morally relevant.

As we have seen, there is considerable disagreement about this. Raymond Frey thinks that only interests$_2$ are morally relevant, whereas Paul Taylor thinks that both interests$_1$ and interests$_2$ are morally relevant. Joel Feinberg thinks that all interests are morally relevant, but this is because he opts for a very restricted notion of 'interests'.

Sparse taxonomies of interests—ones that recognize only one or two kinds of interests—either lump together kinds of interests that should be distinguished, or arbitrarily exclude some kinds of interests. It is for this reason that I have provided a fourfold classification, which plots out all the different ways in which the concept of 'interests' is commonly invoked. We can then ask which of these kinds of interests are morally relevant. It is possible, of course, to have a still richer classification than mine—one that recognizes degrees of consciousness or of self-consciousness, for example. However, such a classification would become unwieldy and therefore less helpful. Moreover, it would pick out differences in *degree* rather than differences in *kind*. As will become evident later, differences in degree can be considered fruitfully after considering what kinds of interests are morally considerable.

WHICH INTERESTS ARE MORALLY CONSIDERABLE?

How does one decide which of the four kinds of interest are morally relevant? This is not a simple matter. It seems as though the arguments for some or other sense of interest are not so much *arguments* for accepting that sense of interest, but rather *explanations* of the *intuition* that that sense of interest is morally relevant. Put another way, it is hard to see how to argue against those whose intuitions differ from one's own. I shall illustrate this by attempting to show why I think that conscious interests are the minimum kind of morally relevant interest. Here is a formalized version of one such argument—an argument that has been advanced in varying forms by a few authors:[11]

(1) To say that an interest is morally relevant is to say that it matters (morally).

(2) If an interest is to matter morally, it must matter to the entity whose interest it is.

(3) For an entity's interest to *matter to it*, there must be something that it is (that is, feels) like to be that entity.

(4) There can only be something that it feels like to be a particular entity if that entity is conscious.

(5) Therefore, only conscious beings can have morally relevant interests.

To avoid misunderstanding, I want to clarify what is meant by saying that an entity's interests *matter* to it. It does not mean that one *wants* what is in one's interests.[12] Instead it means that there is something that it is like to have one's interests served or impeded. Recognizing this enables us to see that there may be an ambiguity in the phrase 'Y has an interest in X'. This phrase can mean either that 'X matters to Y' or that 'Y wants X'. Thus, even if one were to agree with Raymond Frey that animals do

[11] See, for example: Feinberg, Joel, *Rights, Justice and the Bounds of Liberty*, 168; Thompson, Janna, 'A Refutation of Environmental Ethics', *Environmental Ethics*, 12/2 (1990) 147–60 (See, especially, p. 159); Steinbock, Bonnie, *Life Before Birth*, 14; Boonin, David, *A Defense of Abortion* (Cambridge: Cambridge University Press, 2003) 81.

[12] This is the very interpretation that Don Marquis assumes in his critique of Bonnie Steinbock. See his 'Justifying the Rights of Pregnancy: The Interest View', *Criminal Justice Ethics*, 13/1 (1994) 73–4.

not have wants—something I would deny—they could still have morally considerable interests. In other words, one might say that there is a kind of interest intermediate between (a) interest as well-being; and (b) interest as want. It is a kind of interest that involves more than just having a good of one's own (as plants arguably may have), but need not involve as much as a desire that one has self-consciously.

Now the problem with any argument such as the one I have advanced in (1) to (5) above is that the crucial premiss—premiss (3) in this case—is one that will be disputed by those who do not share the intuition embodied in the conclusion. Premiss (3) seems entirely reasonable to me. How, I wonder, can any entity care about its welfare or some aspect of it if there is nothing that it feels like to be such an entity? But the problem is that those who do not share my intuitions can simply deny the premiss. They might claim that there are non-conscious ways in which an entity's welfare can matter to it. (For example, water deprivation may matter to a plant in that it wilts and dies as a result.) Or they might claim that there *is* something that it is like to be a plant (for example), so long as we do not equate 'there is something that it *is* like to be a plant' with 'there is something that it *feels* like to be a plant'. The point can be put another way. To many of us, it seems crucial that one cannot be cruel or kind to plants (because they are not conscious). But others wonder why we should think that only cruelty and kindness are relevant.[13] If we can harm or benefit plants in other ways, why should these other ways not be relevant?

I do not see any decisive argument that could engage and undermine the view of those who think that non-conscious biotic interests are morally relevant. The same is not true, I think, when it comes to the view that functional interests are morally relevant. This view can be decisively rejected on the grounds that functional interests are really interests *of the artefacts* only in a

---

[13] Regan, Tom, 'Feinberg on What Sorts of Beings Can Have Rights?', 490.

figurative sense.[14] I shall not spell out the details of this argument, however, primarily because the question of functional interests can be bypassed in a discussion about abortion, given that zygotes, embryos, and fetuses are never artefacts and thus never have mere functional interests.

Because I cannot give a decisive argument against the moral relevance of non-conscious biotic interests, my argument strategy will be to point out the implications of regarding biotic interests as morally relevant and to show that most if not all pro-lifers do not embrace them.

As I shall show later, fetuses only become conscious quite late in the gestational period. Thus, if conscious interests are the most basic morally relevant interests, fetuses will acquire morally relevant interests only very late. One way of grounding a pro-life argument would be to claim that biotic interests are also morally relevant. However, if biotic interests count morally, a principle of equality would require that equal biotic interests count equally. Thus, it cannot be only *human* biotic interests that are relevant. The interests of plants, bacteria, viruses, and so forth must count as much as the biotic interests of human embryos and preconscious fetuses. But those are implications that very few (if any) pro-lifers will embrace. Consistency requires, then, that they do not ground their view on a claim to the moral relevance of biotic interests. (Of course, this does not mean that there is no other way to support a pro-life position, and I shall consider some other arguments later.)

Those who take biotic interests to be morally relevant do not deny that conscious interests are also relevant. They object only to setting the threshold of relevance above biotic interests. There is another challenge to those who take conscious interests to be the minimum morally relevant interests. This challenge comes from those who would set the threshold above conscious interests—at

[14] Tom Regan ('Feinberg on What Sorts of Beings Can Have Rights?') denies this, but Robert Elliot ('Regan on the Sorts of Beings that Can Have Rights') provides a compelling response.

the level of reflective interests. The implications of this view are also implausible. If only reflective interests count morally, then there can be nothing (directly) wrong with torturing beings that are conscious but not self-conscious—most animals and all human neonates. We can reject the view that *only* reflective interests count.

WHEN DOES CONSCIOUSNESS BEGIN?[15]

None of us can remember when we first became conscious. Therefore, although we were all once fetuses and infants, we cannot settle the question when, in the human developmental process, consciousness begins, by reference to our own recollected experience. To determine when consciousness begins we must treat fetal and infant minds as 'other minds'. Not having first-person access to them, we must infer what they are like from third-person accessible information.

Consider, first, indirect functional evidence of consciousness that is provided by electroencephelography (EEG). The EEG, which records electrical activity of the brain, can provide data about a functional capacity—wakefulness—that is required for consciousness. Wakefulness, it must be stressed, is not to be confused with consciousness itself, at least in neurological parlance. Instead, it is a state of arousal that is to be contrasted with (the various stages of) sleep. Arousal is a state of the ascending arousal system in the brain stem and thalamus. It is not a state of the cerebral cortex. Where the ascending arousal system is connected to an intact functional cortex, its activities bring about changes in the cortex that are discernable clinically and electroencephalographically. While consciousness is supervenient on the function

---

[15] Material in this section is drawn from a paper Michael Benatar and I co-authored: 'A Pain in the Fetus: Ending Confusion about Fetal Pain', *Bioethics*, 15/1 (2001) 57–76. © Blackwell Publishers Ltd.

of the cortex, it is only possible in the wakeful state. In this sense, the brainstem and thalamus only support consciousness indirectly. Since arousal states—wakefulness and sleep—are states of the brain stem and thalamus (even though they usually have cortical consequences), and consciousness is a function of the cortex, wakefulness and consciousness are separable. One can be awake but not conscious. This occurs when the ascending arousal system is in the awake mode, but the cortex is impaired in particular ways. For instance, some patients in persistent vegetative states exhibit wakeful EEG patterns but are unconscious.[16]

Whereas wakefulness is not sufficient for the presence of consciousness, it seems reasonable to assume that consciousness is not possible in the absence of wakefulness. Although sleeping people are sometimes responsive to their environment—that is to say, they can react to stimuli—they are not aware or conscious. If this assumption is correct, then a being that lacks the capacity for wakefulness will also lack the capacity for consciousness. Thus EEGs provide evidence for a condition—wakefulness—without which consciousness is not possible, even though they do not provide evidence of consciousness itself.

Although there are intermittent bursts of (sleep pattern) electroencephalographic activity in fetuses as young as twenty weeks gestation, it is only around thirty weeks that EEGs reveal sleep–wake cycles. In other words, it is only around thirty weeks that the first wakeful states are discernable. At this early stage, it must be emphasized, the EEG patterns for wakefulness and sleep are quite different from those of the adult. In the first few months of postnatal life the fetal EEG pattern gradually gives way to one that much more closely resembles the adult pattern, even though maturation of the EEG continues throughout the first year of life and, to a lesser extent, throughout childhood and adolescence.

---

[16] Multi-Society Task Force on PVS, Medical Aspects of the Persistent Vegetative State, *New England Journal of Medicine*, 330/21 (1994) 1499–508.

There are at least two explanations for the relatively large difference between fetal and adult EEGs. One is that the sort of wakefulness needed for consciousness has not yet developed. The other is that the electroencephalographic differences are a result of the general immaturity (and thus difference) of the fetal nervous system, but suggest nothing about the absence of the neurological function necessary for consciousness. On this view, fetal wakefulness may produce a different EEG, but may still facilitate consciousness. How does one choose between these possible explanations?

One way is to turn from functional evidence for wakefulness to behavioural evidence for consciousness and conscious states such as pain. Consider, for example, the study by Kenneth Craig et al,[17] in which the Neonatal Facial Coding System (NFCS) was used to evaluate the response of *pre-term* neonates to noxious and non-noxious stimuli. Neonates of varying ages were videotaped before, during, and after a heel swab and lancing procedure. The heel swab provides a non-noxious stimulus, whereas the heel lance is a noxious stimulus that would be painful in conscious beings with a mature nervous system. In response to the lance but not the swab, infants older than twenty-eight weeks gestation were found to exhibit a distinct set of facial movements that are also characteristic of term infants and adults subject to painful stimuli. These facial movements include brow lowering, eyes squeezed shut, deepening of the nasolabial furrow, open lips and mouth, and a taut, cupped tongue.[18] The authors of this study also observed that these facial movements varied depending on whether the premature infant was asleep or awake at the time of the lancing. Given that wakefulness facilitates consciousness and thus pain, this observation is noteworthy. In contrast to these striking observations about humans of twenty-eight weeks gestational age,

[17] Craig, K. D., Whitfield, M. F., Grunau, R. V., Linton, J., and Hadjistavropoulos, H. D., 'Pain in the Preterm Neonate: Behavioural and Physiological Indices', *Pain*, 52/3 (1993) 287–99.
[18] Ibid.

infants of twenty-five to twenty-seven weeks gestation did not display a response sufficiently different from baseline.[19]

It is possible, and sceptics of fetal pain might well rush to say, that the facial movements observed in the older pre-term neonates are mere reflexes and do not reflect any (unpleasant) mental state. There is no way decisively to lay such doubts to rest. Nevertheless, the complex and coordinated nature of this behaviour makes it harder to dismiss as a mere reflex.

Reflexive behaviour is that which does not result from a conscious mind. Thus withdrawing from a noxious stimulus is reflexive if it is not a result of a painful feeling. It is not a reflex if it does result from such a feeling. From this, it should not be concluded that the presence of a reflex and the presence of pain are mutually incompatible. Spinal reflexes, for example, can result in the withdrawal of a limb from the source of a noxious stimulus even before the pain-causing impulse has reached the cortex. The withdrawal movement is itself reflex. It does not follow that there is not an accompanying painful sensation, even if that sensation is not the cause of the reflex but rather occurs milliseconds after it. Distinguishing between those behaviours that are both reflexive *and* unaccompanied by painful experiences, and behaviour, whether reflexive or not, that *is* accompanied by pain, can be attempted only by inference. Common sense, derived in part from observing neonates, suggests that humans of late gestational and early post-term age are conscious. The dominant scientific opinion reinforces common sense.

In conclusion, then, there is non-negligible evidence to think that from around twenty-eight to thirty weeks gestational age, fetuses are conscious, at least in some minimal sense. Given the evidence and the gradual nature of the developmental process, it is highly unlikely that the earliest manifestation of consciousness is

[19] The authors of this study caution that the failure to detect these behavioural changes in the younger age group might be an artefact of the small number of infants studied.

fully formed. It is much more likely that the level of consciousness evolves. Indeed, in humans, consciousness also gradually develops into self-consciousness. Thus, conscious interests do not suddenly arise. Instead they emerge gradually, even if not at a constant pace.

INTERESTS IN CONTINUED EXISTENCE

If one only comes into existence in the morally relevant sense at around twenty-eight or thirty weeks gestation, then prior to that stage somebody's coming into existence can still be prevented by means of an abortion. Therefore, if it is better never to come into existence it is better, prior to this time, to be aborted than to be brought to term.

It does not follow from this that abortion any time after around twenty-eight to thirty weeks is (even prima facie) wrong. This is because somebody might grant that a minimally conscious entity may have morally considerable interests, but deny that it has a morally considerable interest in *continued existence*. Thus, it may be argued, it would be prima facie wrong to inflict pain on a conscious (but non-self-conscious) entity, but it may not be wrong to kill it painlessly.

Michael Tooley is one exponent of this view.[20] His argument (part of which resembles the argument of Raymond Frey's that I outlined earlier)[21] can be presented as follows:

(1) The statement 'A has a right to continue to exist as a subject of experiences and other mental states' is roughly synonymous with the statement 'A is a subject of experiences and other mental states, A is capable of desiring to continue to exist as a subject of experiences and other mental states, and if A

[20] Tooley, Michael, 'Abortion and Infanticide', *Philosophy and Public Affairs*, 2/1 (1972) 37–65.
[21] Although I have presented them in the reverse order, Professor Tooley's paper was published before Professor Frey's.

does desire to continue to exist as such an entity, then others are under a prima facie obligation not to prevent him from doing so.'[22]

(2) To have a desire is to want a certain proposition to be true.

(3) To want a proposition to be true one must understand that proposition.

(4) One cannot understand a given proposition unless one has the concepts involved in it.

(5) Therefore, the desires one can have are limited by the concepts one possesses.

(6) Neither a fetus (at any stage of its development) nor a young infant can have concepts of itself as a subject of experiences and other mental states.

(7) Therefore, neither a fetus nor an infant can have a right to continue to exist.

Professor Tooley speaks about when an entity can have a *right* to continued life—and he sometimes speaks about a *serious* right of this kind. Since I am less concerned here with rights than with the (related) concept of interests, I shall discuss his argument as an argument about why fetuses and infants cannot have an interest in continued existence.

There are a number of extremely controversial premises in his argument. First, it is far from clear that an interest in (or right to) continued existence, when unpacked, must make reference to a desire *for continued existence*. It would surely be sufficient that one desires something else that will require continued life in order to be satisfied. Thus if some merely conscious being wants more of the same pleasurable experience it just had, and if that desire and the interest to which it gives rise is morally considerable, this being may have an interest, even if only a weak one, in continued life.

In response to this it might be said that no fetuses or young infants can have *any* desires. But, it is no less controversial that

---

[22] Tooley, Michael, 'Abortion and Infanticide', 46.

an interest in continued existence, when unpacked, must make reference to any *desire*. It is entirely possible that one's interests are served by continued life even if one does not desire it. Professor Tooley does gesture at this problem when he revises his analysis and says that 'an individual's right to X can be violated not only when he desires X, but also when he *would* now desire X were it not for one of the following: (i) he is in an emotionally unbalanced state; (ii) he is temporarily unconscious; (iii) he has been conditioned to desire the absence of X.'[23] These amendments avoid some embarrassing counter-examples. But why, we may wonder, should an additional stipulation not be added?: (iv) he lacks the necessary concepts. What motivates the first three conditions is a sense that continued life is in the interests of those who meet these conditions. But many of us have the same sense that continued life can be in the interests of a conscious entity that lacks the concept of itself as the subject of experiences. If one is going to shoehorn some cases into a desire account one could as easily add another. But a better approach is to say that it is *interests* (of conscious beings) rather than desires that count.

Even if a capacity for desires were necessary, we could still dispute the second premiss—that to have a desire is to want a certain proposition to be true. We can speak quite meaningfully of a baby's desire to have his hunger satiated even if he cannot entertain propositions about hunger and food and the relation between them. When the second premiss collapses, so does the rest of the argument.

Although I think that Professor Tooley's argument should be rejected, his view has a kernel of truth that can be endorsed. To say, as I have suggested, that a minimally conscious entity can have an interest in continued existence is not to say that that interest is anything like as strong as that of a self-conscious entity. Where the interest in continued living is derivative from quite rudimentary

[23] Tooley, Michael, 'Abortion and Infanticide', 48.

interests in further pleasurable experiences, it is much weaker than it becomes when self-consciousness and projects and goals emerge. Then the being is much more invested in its own life and stands to lose much more by dying or being killed. That the earliest interests are weak ones, however, does not mean that they are not interests at all.

One advantage of my view is that moral standing is not something one either has or does not have. There can be varying degrees of it. Given that moral standing is supervenient on other properties, such as consciousness and self-consciousness, and these other properties develop gradually rather than arise suddenly, it makes sense that moral standing be a matter of degree. It would be very odd if it were not wrong at all to kill beings until a certain stage in the developmental process and then it suddenly became *seriously* wrong to kill them.

Given this, we can see that *when* one begins to acquire morally relevant interests is not the only pertinent question in considering whether abortion is morally preferable. It also matters how strong an interest one has in continued existence. Weak and limited interests will be defeated more easily by other considerations. These considerations include the interests of others, but they also include factors like the future quality of life of the person who will develop from the fetus or young infant.

So long as an entity is only minimally invested in its own life, this interest will be more easily defeated by the prospect of future harm. As the interest in existing strengthens, the harms that are required to defeat that interest become more severe. Thus, some late term abortions—after the development of consciousness—and even some instances of infanticide may be morally desirable, if they prevent the continuation of particularly unpleasant existences.

There are two quite famous lines of argument that threaten the view that morally relevant interests, including interests in living, emerge gradually. The first of these is R. M. Hare's Golden

Rule argument and the second is Don Marquis's Future-Like-Ours argument. Both of these arguments aim to show that abortion, even at the earliest stages of pregnancy, is prima facie wrong. I shall consider and reject each of these arguments in turn.

THE GOLDEN RULE

Richard Hare famously employed the 'Golden Rule' to make a prima facie case against abortion.[24] The Golden Rule (in its positive form) says that 'we should do unto others as we would have them do to us.'[25] Logically extending this, he says, yields the rule that 'we should do to others *as we are glad was* done to us.'[26] Given this, since 'we are glad that nobody terminated the pregnancy that resulted in our birth,. . .we are enjoined, *ceteris paribus*, not to terminate any pregnancy which will result in the birth of a person having a life like ours.'[27]

Although much can and has been said about the weaknesses of this argument, I shall discuss those of its flaws that are highlighted by the arguments I have advanced about the harm of coming into existence.

It is not true, of course, that *everybody* is glad not to have been aborted. Professor Hare considers the challenge such people pose to his argument. However, he argues that they must wish that *had* they been glad to have been born, then nobody should have aborted them. The problem with this response is that it assumes that the preference to have been born is the moral touchstone. Had he taken the preference *not* to have been born as the standard, then it could be said that those who *are* glad to have been born

[24] Hare, R. M., 'Abortion and the Golden Rule', *Philosophy and Public Affairs*, 4/3 (1975) 201–22.
[25] Ibid. 208. In its negative form it says that we should *not* do unto others as we would not have them do to us.
[26] Ibid. 208.   [27] Ibid.

must wish that had they not been glad, then somebody should have aborted them. It is obvious that had either kind of person had the opposite preference to the one he does have, the Golden Rule argument would produce the opposite conclusion to the one it does produce when his preference is the way it actually is. Thus Professor's Hare's response to the case of those who are not glad to have been born will not do.

How might we decide which preference—for or against having been born—should prevail? One argument that may be advanced for favouring the preference for having been born is that most fetuses develop into people that have this preference. Thus, working on the presumption that this preference will result is statistically more reliable. However, there are two reasons why, statistical reliability notwithstanding, this preference should not predominate.

First is a principle of caution. Followers of this principle recognize that nobody suffers if one mistakenly presumes a preference not to have been born, but people do suffer if one mistakenly presumes a preference to have been born. Imagine that one presumes that a fetus will develop into somebody who will be glad to have been born. One therefore does not abort the fetus. If one's presumption was mistaken, and this fetus develops into somebody who was not glad to have been born, then there is somebody who suffers (for a lifetime) from one's having made the wrong presumption. Imagine now that one makes the opposite presumption—that the fetus will develop into somebody who will not be glad to have been born. Therefore one aborts that fetus. If this presumption was mistaken, and this fetus would have developed into somebody who would have been glad to have been born, there will be nobody who suffers from the mistaken presumption.

It might be objected that there *is* somebody who suffers from the latter presumption—namely the fetus that is aborted. There are two points that can be made in response. First, this line of reply is not open to Professor Hare. He believes that where an abortion will be performed the 'foetus does not have *now*, at the present moment, properties which are reasons for not killing it, given that it will die in any case before it acquires those properties which ordinary human adults and even children have, and which are our reasons for not killing *them*'.[28] Professor Hare's argument is explicitly about the potential of the fetus rather than any properties it has as a fetus. Secondly, to claim (contrary to Professor Hare) that a fetus does now possess properties that can make it the victim of abortion is to undercut the point of a potentiality argument, such as the Golden Rule argument, against abortion. The entire point of an argument from potentiality is to show that abortion can be wrong even if the fetus does not, as a fetus, have properties that are reasons for not killing it.

A second reason for favouring a preference not to have been born is that coming into existence, as I argued in Chapters 2 and 3, is always a serious harm. If those arguments are sound then people who think that they were benefited by being brought into existence are mistaken and their preference to have come into existence is thus based on a mistaken belief. It would be quite odd to employ a Golden Rule (or Kantian) argument that rests on a mistaken premiss. If a preference is uninformed why should it dictate how we should treat others? Imagine, for example, a widespread preference for having been introduced to cigarettes, which was based on ignorance of the risks of smoking. Employing Professor Hare's rule, people with such a desire could reason: 'I am glad that I was encouraged to smoke, and thus I should encourage others to smoke.' Such reasoning is troubling enough when the preference for having been encouraged to smoke is formulated in the full knowledge of the dangers of smoking. But where the preference is uninformed it cannot even claim to be an (accurate) all things considered judgement and is thus even more troubling.

[28] Hare, R. M., 'A Kantian Approach to Abortion', *Essays on Bioethics* (Oxford: Clarendon Press, 1993) 172.

Similarly, that many people are glad to have come into existence is not a good reason for bringing others into existence, especially where the preference for existence arises from the mistaken belief that one was benefited by being brought into existence.

That the preference for having been born is mistaken lends further support to another (independently) very strong criticism of Professor Hare's argument. It has been noted that the first premiss of his argument—the logical extension of the Golden Rule—is false. There is a difference between being glad that somebody did something for one and thinking that that person was obligated to have done as he did. Not everything that we might wish to be done (or are glad was done) is something that we think should be done (or should have been done). We can wish to be treated in ways that we recognize others are not duty-bound to treat us (or we them).[29] This is true even where one's preferences are not defective. The point is still more powerful when our preferences are uninformed and mistaken.

If, as I have suggested, coming into existence is harmful, and one has not (at the earlier stages of pregnancy) already come into existence in the morally relevant sense, then rational parties would will that they had been aborted. Applying the Golden Rule would then require that they do likewise to others.

A 'FUTURE LIKE OURS'

Don Marquis's argument[30] against abortion starts from the assumption that it is wrong to kill *us*— adult human beings (or at least those adult humans with lives worth continuing, who are innocent of any action that would make it permissible to kill them).

[29] Boonin, David, 'Against the Golden Rule Argument Against Abortion', *Journal of Applied Philosophy*, 14/2 (1997) 187–97.

[30] Marquis, Don, 'Why Abortion is Immoral', *The Journal of Philosophy*, 86/4 (1989) 183–202.

The best explanation of why this is wrong, he says, is that the loss of one's life deprives one of the value of one's future. When one is killed one is deprived of all future pleasures, and of the ability to pursue one's present and future goals and projects. But most fetuses have a valuable future like ours. Thus, concludes Professor Marquis, it must also be wrong to kill these fetuses.

Professor Marquis notes that his argument has a number of virtues. First, it avoids the problem of speciesism. That is to say, it does not claim that human fetal life is valuable merely because it is human. If there are non-human animals who also have valuable futures then it would be wrong to kill them too. And it would not necessarily be wrong to kill those humans, including fetuses, whose future quality of life promises to be so poor that they do not have valuable futures. Secondly, the future-like-ours argument avoids the problems that arise from the view that it is only wrong to kill 'persons'—rational, self-conscious beings. On the future-like-ours argument but not on the personhood criterion, killing of young children and infants is obviously wrong, and for the same reason that killing adults is wrong. Thirdly, the future-like-ours argument does not say that abortion is wrong because it involves the killing of *potential* persons. Such arguments are unable to explain why potential persons are entitled to the same treatment as actual persons. The future-like-ours argument is based on an actual property of the fetus—that it has a future like ours—rather than some potential property.

Professor Marquis considers and rejects two alternatives to his future-like-ours account. According to the 'desire account', what is wrong with killing us is that it thwarts the important desire people have to continue living. But this account, Professor Marquis says, is unable to explain why it is wrong to kill depressives, who have lost the will to live, or those who are sleeping or comatose and therefore cannot be said to have a desire, at the time they are killed, to continue living. Although others have defended a modified desire version of the future-like-ours argument, one that permits abortion,[31] I propose instead to defend what Don Marquis calls a 'discontinuation account'. On this account killing us is wrong because it involves the *discontinuation* of the valuable experiences, activities, and projects of living. Until quite late in pregnancy, as we have seen, fetuses have no experiences, and a fortiori no projects or activities (in any relevant sense).[32] Thus abortion, prior to the development of consciousness, would not be wrong on the discontinuation account.

Don Marquis says that it cannot be the mere discontinuation of experiences that is wrong. If the future experiences will be ones of unmitigated suffering, discontinuation may actually be preferable. Thus, the discontinuation account cannot work unless it refers to the *value* of the experiences that may be discontinued. Moreover, he says, the nature of the immediately past experiences of a person are not relevant. It makes no difference, he says, whether a person *has* been in intolerable pain, *has* been in a coma, or *has* been enjoying a life of value. He concludes that it is *only* the value of the person's future that matters. If that is so, he says, then the discontinuation account must collapse into a future-like-ours account.

But this inference is too quick. A discontinuation account may say that, although the value of the future is necessary for explaining the wrong of killing (those with a valuable future), it is not sufficient. Such an account may hold that only a being with morally relevant interests can have a morally relevant interest in its valuable future. Thus it is the discontinuation of a life of a being that already has morally relevant interests that is wrong. In other words, for killing to be wrong, the future must be a valuable one, but it must also be the future of a being that already counts morally.

Now, Don Marquis might respond that *all* entities with a future like ours do, in virtue of having such a future, have a morally considerable interest—the interest in enjoying that future. But

---

[31] Boonin, David. *A Defense of Abortion*, 62–85.

[32] I add this qualification in case there are some who would want to list 'growing', *in utero* 'kicking' etc., as activities.

why does he think that a (relatively undeveloped) human fetus *now* has such an interest? His answer seems to be that we can by then uniquely identify the entity that will later enjoy that future. This is apparent in his discussion of why contraception is not ruled out by the future-like-ours argument. Contraception prevents futures like ours, but he says that in the case of contraception we cannot (non-arbitrarily) pick out the subject of the deprived future. He considers four possible subjects of harm: (1) some sperm or other; (2) some ovum or other; (3) a sperm and ovum separately; and (4) a sperm and ovum together. He argues that choosing (1) is arbitrary because one could as easily choose (2). And (2) is arbitrary because one could as easily choose (1). Subject (3) cannot be right because then there would be too many futures—that of the sperm and that of the ovum—rather than only the one future of the person who would result were contraception not practised. Finally, he says that (4) cannot be correct. There is no *actual* combination of sperm and ovum. If it is a *possible* combination, we cannot say, of all the possible combinations, which one it is.

I do not think that the morality of abortion or contraception, unlike the issue of when one comes into existence in the biological sense, rests on the identity of an entity. Don Marquis obviously disagrees but because he does so, his view has an odd implication. To see this, imagine that human reproductive biology were a little different from the way it is. Imagine it were the case that instead of sperm and ovum each providing half of the genetic material for the new organism, one of these provided all the DNA and the other provided either only nutrition or an impulse to initiate cell division. If, for instance, a sperm contained all the genetic material and required the ovum only for nutrition,[33] then the relationship between sperm and ovum would be relevantly like the current relationship between zygote and uterus. In that case,

[33] This was the view held by some ancients, such as Aristotle, who thought that the sperm was a homunculus and that the female contribution was only to gestate it.

(1) above could be said to be the victim of contraception, and thus contraception would then be wrong on the future-like-ours argument. Thus the moral issue, on Professor Marquis's view, rests on whether sperm is haploid or diploid.

However, it is hard to see how that can make a difference to whether contraception is morally akin to murder. How, in other words, can mere genetic individuation make all the difference between whether or not it is wrong to prevent a future like ours? If it really is a future like ours that counts, then why should it be the future of *genetically* complete organisms? My alternative proposal, which avoids the odd implication of this, is that what counts is the valuable future of those entities with morally relevant interests. Discontinuing the valuable life of a being with morally relevant interests in that life is (prima facie) wrong.

My account has another advantage over the future-like-ours account. If the value of a future were *all* that counted, then it would be worse to kill a fetus than to kill a thirty-year old. This is because a fetus, all things being equal, would have a longer future, and would therefore be deprived of more. The greater deprivation makes sense when we are comparing the death of a thirty-year old with that of a nonagenarian, where most people take the former to be worse. However, it makes much less sense when comparing the deaths of the fetus and the thirty-year old, where many of us take the latter to be much worse. The best explanation for this is that a fetus has not yet acquired the interest in its own existence that the thirty-year old has. The case of the thirty-year old and the nonagenarian can be explained in one of two ways. It could be that both have equal interests in continued life but the nonagenarian has less life left. Alternatively, in some cases only, it could be that the nonagenarian's interest in living has already begun to decline, perhaps on account of life's becoming worse with advancing age and decrepitude.

There are related ways of explaining intuitions about the relative badness of killing fetuses, young people, and old people. Among these is Jeff McMahan's notion of time-relative interests, which he distinguishes from life interests. The latter 'are concerned with what would be better or worse for oneself as a temporally extended being; they reflect what would be better or worse for one's life as a whole'.[34] Time-relative interests, by contrast, are one's interests at a particular time—that which 'one has egoistic reason to care about'[35] at a particular time. These two kinds of interests are coextensive in so far as identity is the basis for egoistic concern. However, because Professor McMahan (following Professor Parfit)[36] thinks that psychological continuity is more important than identity, life interests and time-relative interests diverge. Arising from each of these interests are competing accounts of the badness of death. Following the 'Life Comparative Account' a death is worse to the extent that the total value of the life it ends is less than it otherwise would have been.[37] On this account the death of the fetus is much worse than the death of the thirty-year old because the total value of the fetus's life is less than the value of the life of one who dies at age thirty. However, on the 'Time Relative Interest Account' the badness of death is assessed in terms of the victim's time-relative interests.[38] Professor McMahan prefers this account, in part because it explains why the death of the thirty-year old is worse than the death of the fetus.[39] The fetus is not prudentially connected to its future self—its future like ours—whereas the thirty-year old is.

CONCLUSIONS

My view that fetuses lack moral standing in the earlier stages of pregnancy is common among advocates of the pro-choice position,

[34] McMahan, Jeff, *The Ethics of Killing: Problems at the Margins of Life* (New York: Oxford University Press, 2002) 80.
[35] Ibid.
[36] Derek Parfit, *Reasons and Persons*, Part 3.
[37] McMahan, Jeff, *The Ethics of Killing*, 105.
[38] Ibid.
[39] Ibid. 105, 165 ff.

although it may be less commonly held that fetuses lack any moral standing for *quite* as long as I have suggested they do. Combining the view that fetuses lack moral standing in the earlier stages of pregnancy with the view that it is always a harm to come into existence turns the prevailing presumptions about abortion on their head. Instead of a presumption in favour of continuing pregnancy, we should adopt a presumption, at least in the earlier stages of pregnancy, against carrying a fetus to term. This is the 'pro-death' view of abortion. On this view, it is not any given abortion (in the earlier stages of pregnancy) that requires justification, but rather any given failure to abort. For such a failure allows somebody to suffer the serious harm of coming into existence.

There may be disagreement about just when during pregnancy a fetus begins to gain moral standing. On the view that consciousness is the appropriate criterion, I have shown that the evidence is that this would be at quite an advanced gestational age. Those who think that the earliest interests in continuing to exist are strong, may think it best, on precautionary grounds, to treat fetuses as having rudimentary moral standing somewhat earlier than that. That would provide a buffer against mistakenly thwarting such an interest. Those who think that the earliest interests in continued existence are weak and that suffering of an ordinary life is very bad, may see no need to regard younger fetuses as having any moral standing. I shall not settle these issues. It seems to me that reasonable people could disagree about the fine evaluative calibrations that would be required to make such judgements. Given that the overwhelming majority of abortions do and could take place well before consciousness arises, I need only conclude that there would be something problematic about willingly or negligently delaying an abortion until the gestation had advanced to the moral grey area.

My argument has not been simply that pregnant women are *entitled* to have an abortion (in the earlier stages). I have argued for the stronger claim that abortion (during these stages) would be *preferable* to carrying the fetus to term. This is *not* the same as arguing that abortions should be forced on people. As I showed in Chapter 4, at least for now we ought to recognize a legal right to reproductive freedom. These arguments apply with at least as much (if not more) force to a freedom not to abort as they do to a freedom to conceive. Thus my conclusions should be viewed as recommendations about how a pregnant woman should make use of the freedom to choose whether or not to abort. I am recommending that she does abort and that she needs excellent reason not to. It should be clear that I do not think that there is any such reason.

The pro-death view should be of interest even to those who do not accept it. One of its valuable features is that it offers a unique challenge to those pro-lifers who reject a legal right to abortion.[40] Whereas a legal pro-choice position does not require a pro-lifer to have an abortion—it allows a choice—a legal pro-life position does prevent a pro-choicer from having an abortion. Those who think that the law should embody the pro-life position might want to ask themselves what they would say about a lobby group that, contrary to my arguments in Chapter 4 but in accordance with pro-lifers' commitment to the restriction of procreative freedom, recommended that the law become pro-death. A legal pro-death policy would require even pro-lifers to have abortions. Faced with this idea, legal pro-lifers might have a newfound interest in the value of choice.

---

[40] Lest it be thought that all pro-lifers, by definition, oppose a legal right to abortion, I should note that one can embrace the pro-life position as the correct moral position, but think that people should nonetheless have a legal right to choose. The distinction is between one's personal moral views and what one thinks the law should say.

6

Population and Extinction

If children were brought into the world by an act of pure reason alone, would the human race continue to exist?

Arthur Schopenhauer[1]

Trillions of conscious beings inhabit our planet. Exponentially more have already lived. How many more lives there still will be remains an open question. Eventually, however, all life will come to an end. Whether this happens sooner or later is one factor that will influence how many more lives there will be. Until then numerous factors will influence the number of beings populating the earth. In the case of humans, the reproductive decisions (or their absence) of individual people, and the population policies (or their absence) of states and international bodies, will play a role.[2]

In this chapter, I shall examine two connected sets of questions. The first set concerns population and the second set concerns extinction. The central question of population—one that has enjoyed considerable philosophical attention—is 'How many people should there be?' By now it should be unsurprising that my

---

[1] Schopenhauer, Arthur, 'On the Sufferings of the World', in *Complete Essays of Schopenhauer*, trans. T. Bailey Saunders, 5 (New York: Wiley Book Company, 1942) 4.

[2] Humans also play a role in deciding how many animals there will be, most obviously in situations in which humans breed animals and in situations in which humans (can) sterilize animals.

answer to this question is 'zero'. Although there are some people who would take this answer to be correct (including some who think that it is obviously so), there are many more who take my answer to be obviously wrong. Part of my aim, therefore, will be to show that my 'zero' answer deserves more serious consideration than it typically receives. To this end, I shall show how it resolves the conundrums of philosophical theory about population.

The central question about extinction, as applied to humans, is 'Is the prospect of human extinction something to be regretted?' I shall answer that although the process of extinction may be regrettable, and although the prospect of human extinction may, in some ways, be bad for us, it would be better, all things considered, if there were no more people (and indeed no more conscious life). A secondary question about extinction is whether, given the fact of future extinction, it would be better if this came earlier or later. Here I shall argue that although very imminent extinction would be worse for us, earlier extinction nonetheless would be better than later extinction. This is because earlier extinction guarantees against the significant harm of future lives that would otherwise be started. I shall show, however, that on some views, the creation of a limited number of new people *may* be justified. If that is so, then although extinction need not come as early as it could it should still come earlier rather than later. Accordingly, even this more modest conclusion is deeply antagonistic to the more common, sentimental view that it would be best, all things being equal, if humans continued to exist for as long as possible.

Although the population and extinction questions are connected, they are distinct. One reason for this is that population size and time-until-extinction need not correlate. Obviously the longer there are humans the more humans there *could* be, but it does not follow that the longer there are humans the more humans there *will* be. Varying the time until extinction is one variable that can influence the number of people, but varying the rate of reproduction is another. Thus, if we imagine extinction occurring about twelve years from now, as a result perhaps of the impact of an asteroid that suddenly makes the planet uninhabitable, there would be, at present rates of reproduction, approximately a further billion people before the end of Homo Sapiens. If the rate of reproduction were halved, the time to extinction could be doubled—the asteroid hits two dozen years from now, rather than half that—without the total number of future people increasing. The relationship between the number of people and the time to extinction need not be coincidental. It could be interactive. Thus, we can imagine circumstances in which making fewer humans ensures that there are humans for a longer time. Perhaps having too many humans would start a war that brought about the end of the species.

OVERPOPULATION

At the time this is being written, there are about 6.3 billion people alive.[3] Very many people think that this is too many—that we already have an overpopulation problem. Others think that unless we do something about population growth (or unless something is done to it), there will very soon be far too many people. Even those who do not think that the population sizes projected for the next century or two would be too big certainly think that there is *some* population size that would be too large. Nobody can reasonably deny that there is some population that would be too large, or, in other words that there *could* be overpopulation.

The notion of *over*population is normative, not descriptive or predictive. There never will be more people than there *could* be,[4] but there may well be more people than there *should* be. But how big a population is overpopulation? This question can be asked of either (a) the cumulative population or (b) a population

---

[3] A billion is 1,000,000,000.
[4] However, there may be more people than there could be *for very long*.

at any given time. The latter question—how many people may there be at any given time?—is the usual one. This is because the number of people living at any one time can impact on the welfare of those (and later) people,[5] or (some environmentalists would argue) impact on the planet. Anthropocentrically, there may not be enough food to go around, or the world may simply become too crowded. Environmentally, the ecological 'footprint' of a very large human population may be too great.[6] Thus the usual concern is to avoid having too many people around at one time or within some specified period. That is a reasonable concern. However, as I have indicated, we can also ask the population question about the cumulative population—how many people may there be throughout time?[7] In so far as most people can make sense of this question, it is a function of the concurrent population, the (possible) duration of humanity, and the circumstances of each period of humanity. In other words, their answer to the question 'How many people may there be throughout time?' is calculated by summing,[8] for every consecutive period of humanity's possible duration, the answers to the question 'How many people may there be within this period?' However, as I shall show, the question about cumulative population size can be asked and answered in other ways.

My argument that coming into existence is always a great harm, implies a radical answer to the population question (in both of its forms). It suggests that a cumulative population numbering only one person would have been overpopulation. This is not because there would have been too many people for the earth, or too many people to be sustained by the earth. Instead it is because coming

[5] See, for example, Kates, Carol A., 'Reproductive Liberty and Overpopulation', *Environmental Values*, 13 (2004) 51–79.

[6] The ecological footprint is obviously not only a function of population size, but also of the per capita impact. A small human population can make a big impact on the environment.

[7] Those who ask this question often phrase this question as follows: 'How many people should there *ever* be?' (e.g., Derek Parfit, *Reasons and Persons*, 381).

[8] In ways that take account of overlapping populations.

into existence is a serious harm—and one such serious harm would have been one too many.

In fact, however, by my standards there have been already billions too many humans. Determining how many billions is a difficult matter. When, for example, do we start counting? To know how many humans there have been we need to know for how long there have been humans, and there is obvious scientific disagreement, within a certain range, about this.[9] We also need to know, but do not know, how many humans there were for much of human history. However, on one influential assessment there have been well in excess of 106 billion people.[10] Nearly 6 per cent of those people are alive today.[11] The early human population was small. One author suggests that a 'combination of ecological reasoning and anthropological observation indicates that the savannahs of eastern and southern Africa [where humans originated] would have supported approximately 50,000 early humans.'[12] By about 10,000 years ago and the advent of agriculture, the human population had increased to an estimated 5 million.[13] It grew to 500 million by the dawn of the industrial revolution.[14] Growth of the world human population sped up considerably since then. It took over a century (1804–1927) to increase from 1 billion to 2 billion, but each subsequent billion took less and less time—33 years for the third billion in 1960, 14 years for the fourth billion in 1974, 13 years for the fifth billion in 1987, and 12 years for the sixth billion in 1999.[15]

[9] I here ignore the obviously false view of the crudest creationists that there have only been humans for close on 6,000 years.

[10] Carl Haub, 'How Many People Have Ever Lived on Earth?', originally published in *Population Today* in February 1995. My statistic comes from an updated version on the web: <http://www.prb.org/Content/ContentGroups/PTarticle/Oct-Dec02/How_Many_People_Have_Ever_Lived_on_Earth_.htm> (accessed 5 October 2004).

[11] Ibid.

[12] McMichael, Anthony, *Human Frontiers, Environments and Disease* (Cambridge: Cambridge University Press, 2001) 188.

[13] Ibid.

[14] Ibid.

[15] <http://www.peopleandplanet.net> (accessed 5 October 2004).

Although it would have been better had none of the more than 106 billion people come into existence, these people (among whom you and I are included) can no longer be prevented. For this reason, many might wish to focus on the question how many *more* people there may be—in the cumulative sense, rather than at some specified time in the future. The ideal answer here is again 'zero', although that ideal is being violated about every second.[16]

SOLVING PROBLEMS IN MORAL THEORY ABOUT POPULATION

My argument that coming into existence is always a serious harm, if accepted, provides an interesting solution to a set of problems in moral theory about population. Some authors have seen the view that there should be no more people not as a solution to such problems, but instead as another of the problems. That, however, is because they have considered only the conclusion that there should be no more people rather than the argument for this conclusion. In other words, as I shall show, it has been noted that some moral theories imply that there should be no more people, and then the theory has been rejected on the grounds that it has such an (allegedly outrageous) implication. However, now that I have given an independent argument for the view that there should be no more people, it should be seen that it is not a weakness but rather a strength of a moral theory that it has this implication.

Professor Parfit's population problems

The *locus classicus* of moral theorizing about population is Part 4 of Derek Parfit's *Reasons and Persons*. His discussion is long

---

[16] At present the human population increases by 200,000 people a day (and this is *after* the daily deaths are counted).

and complex and thus not every feature of it can be presented here. However, I shall provide a brief outline of his central arguments before showing what bearing my arguments have on his discussion.

Professor Parfit discusses the non-identity problem. This problem, it will be recalled from my discussion in Chapter 2, arises where the only alternative to bringing about a poor quality life is not bringing about that life at all. The non-identity problem is the problem of explaining the common judgement that starting such a life is wrong. Professor Parfit argues that what he calls 'person-affecting' views of morality cannot explain why starting such a life is wrong. A person-affecting view is one that morally assesses an action in terms of how it affects people. In his first statement of the person-affecting view, Professor Parfit describes it as the view that 'it is bad if people are affected for the worse.'[17] Such a view, he says, cannot solve the non-identity problem because in non-identity cases those who are brought into existence cannot be *worse* off than they would otherwise have been, because they would not otherwise have been.

It is the person-affecting view's alleged inability to solve the non-identity problem that sets Professor Parfit off on his hunt for the elusive Theory X, a theory that must solve the non-identity problem while avoiding other problems generated along the way. Because he believes that person-affecting views cannot solve the non-identity problem, he considers the alternative—impersonal views. Whereas person-affecting views maintain that something can only be bad if it is worse for somebody, impersonal views are not concerned about the effects on particular people. Instead they examine outcomes more impersonally. If people's lives go better in one possible outcome than the other, then the better outcome is to be preferred even though nobody is better off in that scenario.

[17] Parfit, Derek, *Reasons and Persons*, 370.

This view can explain why it is wrong to bring into existence a person who will have a poor quality life. It is wrong because that outcome is worse than the alternative outcome in which that person is not brought into existence. It does not matter, on the impersonal view, that the person brought into existence is not worse off than he would otherwise have been. It is enough that the outcome in which he comes into existence is worse (impersonally) than the outcome in which he does not come into existence. In other words, an impersonal view can solve the non-identity problem.

The impersonal view, however, cannot be Theory X, because although it solves the non-identity problem, it has serious problems of its own. To understand why this is so, we must distinguish two kinds of impersonal view:

Impersonal Total View:
'If other things are equal, the best outcome is the one in which there would be the greatest quantity of whatever makes life worth living.'[18]
Impersonal Average View:
'If other things are equal, the best outcome is the one in which people's lives go, on average, best.'[19]

Consider first the problem with the impersonal total view. On this view, a smaller population with a higher quality of life is worse than a larger population with a smaller quality of life so long as there are enough extra people in the larger population to outweigh the lower quality of life. Derek Parfit represents these two worlds as shown in Figure 6.1.[20]

In these diagrams, the width of the bar corresponds to the number of people and the height to the quality of life. The A-population is very small but has a high quality of life. The Z-population is very

---

[18] Parfit, Derek, *Reasons and Persons*, 387.   [19] Ibid. 386.
[20] Ibid. 388. He represents a range of intermediate worlds as well. The components of the diagram included here are reproduced by permission of Oxford University Press.

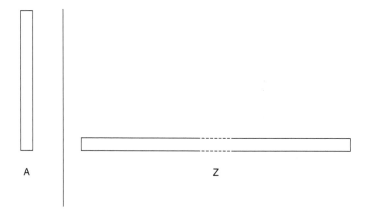

Figure 6.1.

large, but has a low quality of life. Indeed, life in Z is barely worth living. However, the total amount of goodness in Z is greater than the total amount of goodness in A. Thus, Z is better, according to the impersonal total view. This is so even though the people in the more populous world lead lives of a lower quality. The conclusion that Z is better than A, Derek Parfit rightly suggests, is repugnant. Hence he terms it the 'Repugnant Conclusion'.[21]

The impersonal average view avoids the Repugnant Conclusion because that view requires that the total good in a world be divided by the number of people in the world, in order to determine the average well-being. In the more populous world, the average quality of life is much, much lower. It is worse, therefore, than the less populous world.

[21] Ibid. 388. Not everybody views this conclusion as repugnant. Torbjörn Tännsjö, for example, thinks that most people lead lives that are only just worth living. When we rise above this level we do so only briefly. If people recognized that the quality of life in Z was the same quality as their lives, they would not accept that the Repugnant Conclusion really is repugnant. (See his *Hedonistic Utilitarianism* (Edinburgh: Edinburgh University Press, 1998) 161–2. See also his 'Doom Soon?', *Inquiry*, 40/2, (1997) 250–1.) Although I shall not engage Professor Tännsjö's views directly, arguments I have already advanced and others I shall still provide show what is wrong with his argument.

Although the impersonal average view also solves the non-identity problem, it too cannot be Theory X, for it faces other problems. To show why this is the case, Derek Parfit asks us to imagine another two worlds. In the first world everybody had a very high quality of life. In the second world, in addition to all these people with their same high quality of life there are additional people who, although not quite as well off, nonetheless have lives that are well worth living. These sorts of cases, Derek Parfit calls 'Mere Addition'. More specifically, mere addition occurs 'when, in one of two outcomes, there exist extra people (1) who have lives worth living, (2) who affect no one else, and (3) whose existence does not involve social injustice'.[22]

Now the impersonal average view says that the second world is worse, because the average quality of life is lower. It is made lower by the mere addition of extra people who, although happy, are not quite as happy as the original people are. Derek Parfit takes this to be implausible. It would entail, he says, that it would be worse if *in addition* to Adam and Eve leading blissful lives, there were a billion extra people who lived lives of slightly lower quality. The impersonal average view also entails, he says, that whether it is wrong to have any given child depends on facts about the quality of all previous lives. Thus, if 'the ancient Egyptians had a very high quality of life, it is more likely to be bad to have a child now'.[23] But, says Professor Parfit, 'research in Egyptology cannot be relevant to our decision whether to have children.'[24] Accordingly, he takes the impersonal average view to be implausible.

Why anti-natalism is compatible with Theory X

If my arguments are taken seriously, then a number of Professor Parfit's problems can be overcome. First, I argued in Chapter 2 that the non-identity problem can be solved. One way in which I

[22] Parfit, Derek, *Reasons and Persons*, 420.
[23] Ibid.   [24] Ibid.

said this might be done is by employing Joel Feinberg's argument that coming into existence *can* be worse for that person than never existing. Alternatively, I argued, we can say that even if coming into existence is not *worse*, it may still be *bad* for the person who comes into existence. Since the alternative is *not bad* we can say that the person is thereby harmed. This alternative argument may seem inadequate if the person-affecting view is understood, as I have suggested so far, as the view that something 'is bad if people are affected for the *worse*'.[25] However, that first formulation of Derek Parfit's is more restrictive than it need be. When he later distinguishes two kinds of person-affecting principles—the narrow and the wide—he describes one of them as follows:

The Narrow Person-Affecting View:
'An outcome is worse for people (in the narrow sense) if the occurrence of X rather than Y would be either worse, *or bad*, for the X-people.'[26]

The reason why Professor Parfit thinks that addition of an 'or bad' clause cannot solve the non-identity problem is that he thinks it is not bad for people to come into existence so long as they have a life worth living. However, I have explicated an ambiguity in the phrase 'a life worth living', noting that it might mean either 'a life worth starting' or 'a life worth continuing'. Keeping this distinction in mind and considering the argument that coming into existence is always a harm, it follows that no lives are worth starting (even if some lives are worth continuing). Thus coming into existence is always bad for a person even if one thinks that it is not worse for that person.

Given that a person-affecting view is indeed able to solve the non-identity problem, there is no need to appeal to an impersonal view to solve it. Some may see my arguments as bolstering the case against the impersonal view. The repugnant conclusion, for

[25] Ibid. 370 (emphasis added).
[26] Ibid. 395 (emphasis added).

example, is even more repugnant on my view than it is on the view that, all things being equal, it is good to have extra lives. On my view, adding extra lives is worse (because it increases the number of people harmed), and especially when those extra lives are barely worth continuing. The more populous world with poorer quality lives is, in *every* way, worse than the less populous world with better quality lives.

Others might suggest that if the impersonal total view takes account of my argument it can avoid the repugnant conclusion. My argument may be seen to explain that the repugnant conclusion arises because of the mistaken assumption that it is good to have extra lives that are worth continuing. The impersonal total view can be revised to avoid both this mistake and the resultant conclusion. One way in which this can be done is to restrict the scope of the impersonal total view in such a way that it applies only to people who do exist or will anyway exist and not to questions about how many people should exist. In other words, it can be seen as a principle to maximize the happiness of the existent, but not to affect the number of existers. This revision, however, comes at an obvious cost. The revised view ceases to provide guidance on how many people there should be.

My arguments also shed some light on the impersonal average view. This view, it will be recalled, faces the (alleged) problem of mere addition.[27] That is to say, the impersonal average view says that we should not add extra lives if they lower the average well-being of all humans who have ever lived. The implication that additional lives 'worth living'—read 'worth continuing'—should not be added is taken to be implausible. My arguments, however, show that it is not. If no lives are worth starting, it is not a defect

[27] Derek Parfit goes on to describe not merely a Mere Addition *problem*, but a Mere Addition *paradox*. For the sake of simplicity, I shall not venture on to discuss the paradox. My comments on the Mere Addition problem can be extrapolated to the paradox. For those familiar with the paradox, my solution is to deny that Derek Parfit's A+ is not worse than A. On my view A+ is definitely worse than A, because it involves extra lives (and thus extra harm).

in a theory that it precludes adding new lives that are not worth starting, even if those lives would be worth continuing. It would indeed have been better if no people had been added to the Edenic lives of Adam and Eve.

However, this is not to support the impersonal average view, for on this view we would be obliged to start new lives if it would raise the average quality of life of all people who have every lived. This is at odds with my conclusion and it would still imply that Egyptology is relevant to our procreative decisions. As with the impersonal total view, the impersonal average view is concerned about how much good there is and not with how well off people are. Both impersonal views make the mistake of valuing people only to the extent that they increase (total or average) happiness. They mistakenly assume that the value of happiness is primary and the value of persons is derivative from this. However, as I noted in Chapter 2, it is not the case that people are valuable because they add extra happiness. Instead extra happiness is valuable because it is good for people—because it makes people's lives go better.

The total and average impersonal views can be revised in a way that this mistake does no harm. This is another way of avoiding their respective problems—the repugnant conclusion and the mere addition problem. Under this revision, the impersonal views seek not the greatest total or average happiness but rather the smallest total or average unhappiness. In other words, the revised impersonal views seek to minimize the total or average unhappiness. This way of revising the impersonal views has two advantages. First, it preserves the impersonal view's ability to provide guidance on how many people there should be. Secondly, it generates the conclusion for which I have argued—namely that the ideal population size is 'zero'. The way to minimize unhappiness is for there to be no people (or other conscious beings). The lowest total unhappiness and the lowest average unhappiness are both zero unhappiness, and zero unhappiness, at least in the real world, is achieved by having zero people.

Those who wish, at this point, to resurrect the repugnant conclusion and mere addition problems by imagining a world in which no lives contain any bad but differ only in how much good they contain face a number of problems. First, it is not clear that we can even make sense of such a world, given the interaction between the good and bad in a life. As I showed in Chapter 3, a life that contained very little good would have to contain some bad—namely the tedium of long stretches of absent goods. The only way this could be avoided would be if the life's duration were shortened, but the shortening of life is another bad.

If we assume that this problem can be overcome, then a second one arises. Consider first the repugnant conclusion. What is repugnant about the repugnant conclusion is the suggestion (entailed by the impersonal total view) that a world filled with lives barely worth living is better than a world containing many fewer lives of much greater quality. But how could lives be barely worth living (read 'worth continuing') if they contained no bad—and the absence of more good were not bad? In other words, how can a life containing only good and no bad be barely worth continuing? If the lives in Z are actually quite well worth living then preferring Z over A is no longer repugnant (even if one thinks that it is still mistaken).

Consider mere addition next. It is true that if future possible lives were known to contain no bad, even the unhappiness-minimizing version of the impersonal average view could not rule out mere addition. However, the question is whether this would be problematic. Much of the reason why mere addition is seen as a problem is that the average impersonal view's rejection of mere addition runs counter to an implicit assumption that it is good to have extra lives that are worth living. The average impersonal view says that it can be bad to have extra lives that are worth living (if these extra lives lower average well-being). Where lives contain some bad I have shown that my argument says that the impersonal average view is right to reject mere addition. Although my argument does not show that the impersonal average view is right to reject mere addition in cases where the extra lives contain no bad, it helps nevertheless to overcome the problem. Remember that, following my argument in Chapter 2, a (hypothetical) life that contains some good but no bad is not worse than never existing—but neither is it any better than never existing. Following my argument, there is no way to choose between (a) never existing and (b) coming into existence with a life that contains no bad whatsoever. This makes the impersonal average view's judgement of mere addition less implausible. If it is better to have extra lives worth living and the impersonal average view suggests that it is worse, then there is a serious problem. However, if on one criterion, there is no way of choosing in favour of or against mere addition, and the impersonal average view suggests we choose against, then there need not be any contradiction. The impersonal average view can be seen as layering a further (impersonal) condition upon a judgement that mere addition is neither better nor worse for those who are added.

In addition to solving the non-identity problem and avoiding both the repugnant conclusion and the mere addition problem, my argument that coming into existence is always a harm also explains 'The Asymmetry':

While it would be wrong to have a child that would have a life not worth continuing, there is no moral reason to have a child that would have a life well worth continuing.[28]

Given that coming into existence is always a harm (even if that life would be worth continuing), there can never be a moral reason to have a child—or, at least, no all-things-considered moral reason.

[28] This wording of the asymmetry is an adaptation of Derek Parfit's formulation (p. 391), which would require familiarity with his 'Wretched Child' and 'Happy Child' examples. My formulation also avoids problems with the ambiguity in the phrase 'a life worth living'.

(There may be a *pro tanto* reason[29]—such as the interest of the prospective parents.)

My argument that coming into existence is always a harm thus does much of what Derek Parfit says that Theory X needs to do. It

1. solves the non-identity problem;
2. avoids the repugnant conclusion;
3. avoids the mere addition problem; and
4. explains the asymmetry.

This is not to suggest that my view is Theory X. Mine is an argument only about whether there should be more people, whereas Theory X is a general theory about morality that can also deal satisfactorily with population questions. However, the fact that my argument, unlike so many others, appears compatible with Theory X in all these ways provides some further grounds for taking my argument seriously, even though for many people its conclusion is radically counter-intuitive.

Contractarianism

Whether contractarianism[30] could provide guidance about how many people there should be is a matter of dispute. Derek Parfit thinks that it cannot fulfil this function.

On the ideal contractarian view, principles of justice are chosen in what John Rawls calls the 'original position'—a hypothetical position in which impartiality is ensured by denying parties in the position knowledge of particular facts about themselves. The

[29] This is Shelly Kagan's term. By it he means a reason that 'has genuine weight, but nonetheless may be outweighed by other considerations'. He distinguishes it from the more commonly used '*prima facie* reason', which he takes to 'involve an epistemological qualification' which '*appears* to be a reason, but may actually not be a reason at all, or may not have weight in all cases it appears to'. (*The Limits of Morality* (Oxford: Clarendon Press, 1989) 17.)

[30] Here I consider only ideal contractarianism—the view that morality consists in those principles that would be chosen under some ideal set of circumstances—as this is the dominant and most plausible version of contractarianism.

problem, however, says Derek Parfit, is that parties in the original position must know that they exist. But to assume, when choosing principles that affect future people, that we shall certainly exist, he says, 'is like assuming, when choosing a principle that would disadvantage women, that we shall certainly be men'.[31] This is a problem because it is essential to ideal contractarianism 'that we do not know whether we would bear the brunt of some chosen principle'.[32]

Now the problem with this objection to contractarianism is that the analogy does not hold, and it does not hold because only existers can 'bear the brunt' of any principle. A principle that results in some possible people never becoming actual does not impose any costs on those people. Nobody is disadvantaged by not coming into existence. Rivka Weinberg makes the same point in a different way. She says that 'existence is not a distributable benefit' and thus neither 'people in general nor individuals in particular will be disadvantaged by the assumption of an existent perspective'.[33]

Those who are unsatisfied with this response might wish to consider whether the original position could be altered in such a way that parties to it do not know whether they will exist. Derek Parfit thinks that such a change cannot be made. This, he says, is because while we 'can imagine a different possible history, in which we never existed . . . we cannot assume that, in the actual history of the world, it might be true that we never exist'.[34] But it is not clear to me why this explains why possible people cannot be parties to the original position. Why must parties in the original position be people in 'the actual history of the world'? Why can we not imagine instead that they are possible people? Some may object that it is metaphysically too fanciful to think of possible people inhabiting an original position. However, the whole point about

---

[31] Parfit, Derek, *Reasons and Persons*, 392.   [32] Ibid.
[33] Weinberg, Rivka M., 'Procreative Justice: A Contractualist Account', *Public Affairs Quarterly*, 16/4 (2002) 408.
[34] Parfit, Derek, *Reasons and Persons*, 392.

the original position is that it is a hypothetical position, not an actual one. Why might we not imagine hypothetical people inhabiting a hypothetical position? Professor Rawls's theory is intended to be 'political not metaphysical'[35] and the original position, he emphasized, is but an expository device to determine fair principles of justice. These are principles that it would be rational to adopt were we truly impartial.

What size population would be produced by principles chosen by parties in the original position? This obviously depends on a variety of features of the original position. If we admit possible people to the original position, but hold constant all other features of that position, as Professor Rawls describes it, we find that the chosen principles would produce my ideal population—zero. Professor Rawls says that parties to the original position would maximize the position of the worst off—that is, they would maximize the minimum—so-called 'maximin'. Many writers agree that when applied to questions of population size, this would imply that there should be no people.[36] This is because, as long as procreation continues, some of those people who are brought into being will lead lives that are not worth living (read 'worth continuing'). The only way to improve their position is not to bring such people into existence, and the only way to guarantee that such people are not brought into existence is not to bring anybody into existence.

Michael Bayles thinks that maximin produces this conclusion only if it is utilities that are being distributed. If it is primary goods—goods that are needed to secure all other goods—he says that the opposite conclusion would be produced. He says that the 'worst off are the nonexistent, for they do not receive any primary

---

[35] Rawls, John, 'Justice as Fairness: Political not Metaphysical', *Philosophy and Public Affairs*, 14/3 (1985).
[36] Rivka Weinberg, for example, says that 'Maxi-Min would lead to a procreative ban since no procreation is better than being born with an incurable disease that makes life not worth living.' ('Procreative Justice: A Contractualist Account', 415.)

goods. The next worse off class consists of those who may or may not exist, and if they exist they will receive some primary goods. Consequently one should bring as many people as possible into existence.'[37]

Underlying this line of reasoning is the mistaken assumption that the non-existent can be badly off on account of absent goods. However, we saw in Chapter 2 (Fig. 2.1, quadrant 4) that absent goods are not bad if there is nobody who is deprived by their absence. Thus the non-existent are not the worst off. Indeed, my argument shows that existers are always worse off on account of existing and thus maximin does indeed suggest that zero population is the optimum size.

Those who have seen this implication of maximin for population questions have taken it to be grounds for rejecting maximin. That is, they take the implication to be a *reductio ad absurdum* of maximin. My arguments suggest that that dismissal is mistaken.[38] Those who reject the implication of maximin often think that it matters what the probability of a bad outcome is, and thus parties in the original position should be able to reason probabilistically. Professor Rawls imposes a condition on the original position that prevents this. My arguments show that, for population questions, it makes no difference whether parties in the original position may reason probabilistically or not. This is because it is *always* very bad to come into existence. Thus the probability of a bad outcome is one hundred per cent. How bad the outcome is—very, very, very bad or just very bad—is a matter of probability. However, that does not matter in the current context, given that one already knows that any outcome in which one exists holds no advantages for oneself over an outcome in which one does not. Thus even

[37] Bayles, Michael, *Morality and Population Policy* (University of Alabama Press, 1980) 117.

[38] However, more can be said about this. The reductio argument is advanced not only against maximin but also against my conclusion that coming into existence is always a harm. I shall say more about this in the opening section of Chapter 7.

those who think that (a) probabilities should be taken into account, (b) the interests of parents and children should be balanced, and (c) procreation should be permitted 'only when it would not be irrational'[39] will be led to the same conclusion as those who choose to maximin. If my argument is right, it is always irrational to prefer to come into existence. Rational impartial parties would choose not to exist and the upshot of this is zero population.

PHASED EXTINCTION

I have shown that my arguments help to solve a number of notorious problems in moral theory about population. Indeed a number of these problems arise precisely because of a failure to recognize that coming into existence is always a serious harm. However, although my view helps to solve those population problems that are usually discussed, it faces other problems of its own. I turn now to consider these and to show how they might be solved.

My answer to the question 'How many people should there be?' is 'zero'. That is to say, I do not think that there should ever have been any people. Given that there have been people, I do not think that there should be any more. But this 'zero' answer, I said earlier, is an ideal answer. Do any features of the non-ideal real world permit a less austere answer?

When decreasing population decreases quality of life

The population problems that we have looked at so far have involved creating extra people. The non-identity problem was a problem of explaining why creating some person was wrong. The repugnant conclusion arises in cases where adding extra lives

---

[39] 'Procreative Justice: A Contractualist Account', 420.

lowers the quality of life. The mere addition problem arises from the 'mere addition' of extra people who have 'lives worth living'. My arguments solve these problems by showing that none of these extra people should be brought about.

The problems my argument generates arise not from the creation of extra people but rather from failing to create extra people. For many people the extinction that would result from universal acceptance of my view is the biggest such problem. Later in this chapter I shall argue against this view, showing that there is nothing regrettable about some future state in which there are no more people. Instead the population problem that I believe poses a greater challenge is the path to extinction rather than extinction itself.

In our heavily populated world, we are accustomed to thinking of increased population being correlated with decreased quality of life. However, it is also possible, in other circumstances, for a decrease in population to be correlated with decreased quality of life. This can occur in one of two related ways. If a population shrinks too rapidly and it does so as result of a lower birth rate (rather than a higher death rate, particularly of older people), quality of life can be reduced because a larger proportion of the population is non-productive on account of its advanced age. In such cases, the younger adult people cannot produce enough to sustain the previous quality of life for the entire population. In such cases, it is not the absolute size of the reduced population that causes the lower quality of life. Instead it is the ratio of young to old people that results from a population reduction induced by a falling birth rate.

The other, related way in which decreasing population can decrease quality of life is not when one generation is merely relatively less populous than the one before it, but rather when the size of a new generation falls beneath one of a number of thresholds. In such cases, the absolute (and not merely the relative) size of the population is so small that quality of life is decreased. Consider an extreme case, around the lowest threshold. Adam and Eve are the only people who ever live. (Cain, Abel, and Seth are never born.) Adam dies and widowed Eve is left without any human company.[40] Eve's quality of life is reduced not because the human population is now fifty per cent of what it was before, but because it has fallen beneath some threshold—in this case the threshold necessary for company. Had she had children she would at least have had some human company after Adam's death.

Bringing people into existence always inflicts serious harm on those people. However, in some situations failing to bring people into existence can make the lives of existent people a lot worse than they would otherwise have been. That is cause for concern. However, we need to avoid a protracted regress in which more and more harm is done by the addition of successive new generations in order to prevent extra harm to existing people. Thus, the creation of new generations could only possibly be acceptable, on my view, if it were aimed at phasing out people.

Unless humanity ends suddenly, the final people whether they exist sooner or later, will likely suffer much.[41] There is some sense in making sure that fewer people suffer this fate. This can be done by steadily reducing the number of people. I am under no illusions. Although humans may voluntarily seek to reduce their number, they will never, under current circumstances, do so with the intention of moving towards extinction. Thus, in considering the question of phased extinction from a large population base, I am not discussing what will ever happen but only what should happen or what it would be best to have happen. Put another way, I am discussing the theoretical implications and applications of my views.

Imagine two possible populations in the near future, as represented in Figure 6.2.

---

[40] In any event, she has fallen out with the snake.

[41] Given that procreators are not deterred from procreating by the suffering that their own children will endure, it should be unsurprising that they are not deterred by the suffering of the final people in the more distant future. However if it transpires that the suffering of the final people is great enough, those people might wish that their parents and earlier ancestors had created new people.

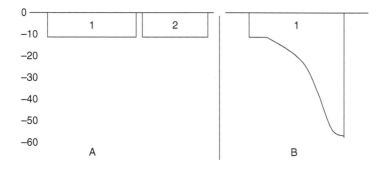

Figure 6.2.

As in Figure 6.1, the width (that is, along the horizontal axis) of 1 and 2 represents population size, with wider (and additional) shapes representing more people. A is a population that would exist if procreation continued, but at about seventy-five per cent of replacement rate. B is the population that would exist if we ceased procreation with immediate effect. In both futures, all lives are beneath the zero quality level—by which I mean the level just above which a life becomes worth starting (and not the level just above which life becomes worth continuing). This is a departure from Derek Parfit's representation in Figure 6.1. Although he does not think that all lives on the positive scale are worth living (and thus the baseline of his bars is not the level at which lives become worth living),[42] his general assumption is that some lives are worth living and all these lives have net positive value. Given my views, all lives are either more bad or less bad, not more good or less good. This is why I use the negative scale beneath the zero quality level. The worse the quality of life the lower it extends on the vertical axis.

The 1-people are the same people in A and B. In A, the 1-people are those who exist before the 2-people are brought into existence.

---

[42] See his reference to the 'Bad Level' in *Reasons and Persons*, 432–3.

Bringing the 2-people into existence makes the lives of the already existent people much less bad than they would otherwise be. The absence of the 2-people in B, makes the lives of the already existent people much worse. But it does not do so for all the 1-people in B. This is because some of them will die before the impact of the absence of 2-people can be felt. The extent of the harm to the 2-people is determined by how bad their lives are. This is because the harm of coming into existence is not distinct from the bad in the life that is started. In other words, how bad a life actually is, is the same as how bad it is to come into existence with such a life. In Figure 6.2 I assume, for the sake of simplicity, that the new lives will have the same quality as the previous ones—that is, that they will be as bad (but not worse) than the lives of the 1-people in A. This assumes that the 2-people are not the final people. If they were the final people, many of them would lead lives much worse than the 1-people in A, which would instead resemble the lives of the 1-people in B. Any full assessment of the ethics of phased extinction would have to take into account the harms of all generations up to and including the final people. Here I simplify the question by focusing only on one new generation.

On the view that the 2-people are harmed by being brought into existence, may they nonetheless be brought into existence given the extent to which their existence makes the lives of some of the 1-people less bad? More generally, my anti-natalist view must face the following questions:

1. May we ever create new lives in order to improve the quality of existent lives?
2. If so, under what conditions may we do so?

Reducing population to zero

These questions cannot be answered by the narrow person-affecting view. This, it will be recalled, is the view that:

'An outcome is worse for people (in the narrow sense) if the occurrence of X rather than Y would be either worse, or bad, for the X-people.'[43]

I showed that this view *can* solve the non-identity problem. The narrow person-affecting view can also show why world B in Figure 6.2 is worse for the 1-people and why world A is worse for the 2-people. However, the narrow person-affecting view cannot answer the two questions before us now. It provides no guidance on whether we may ever inflict harm by bringing new people into existence if that will reduce the harm of those who already exist and, if so, under what conditions we may do so. The narrow person-affecting view cannot tell us whether we may bring the 2-people into existence if that will reduce the harm of (many of) the 1-people.

The wide person-affecting view, by contrast, is able to answer our two questions and can say whether A is worse than B. However, as I shall show, it cannot answer these questions in a way that takes seriously the view that coming into existence is always a serious harm.

The Wide Person-Affecting View:
'An outcome is worse for people (in the wide sense) if the occurrence of X would be less good for the X-people than the occurrence of Y would be for the Y-people.'[44]

The wide person-affecting view says that we may start new lives in order to improve the quality of existent lives if the harm suffered by existing people in the absence of new people would be greater than the harm done to the new people.

But under what conditions can the one harm be said to be greater than the other? How does one make such comparisons? Derek Parfit suggests two versions of the wide person-affecting view, each of which spells out different ways of making the comparison:

[43] Parfit, Derek, *Reasons and Persons*, 395.
[44] Ibid. 396.

Wide Total Person-Affecting View:

> An outcome is worse for people 'if the *total net benefit* given to the X-people by the occurrence of X would be less than the total net benefit given to the Y-people by the occurrence of Y'.[45]

Wide Average Person-Affecting View:

> An outcome X is worse for people 'if the *average net benefit per person* given to the X-people by the occurrence of X would be less than the average net benefit per person given to the Y-people by the occurrence of Y'.[46]

Given that everybody, on my view, is harmed, it may be better to express these principles in terms of 'harms' rather than 'benefits' — that is negatively rather than positively:

Negative Wide Total Person-Affecting View:

> An outcome is worse for people if the *total net harm* to the X-people by the occurrence of X would be greater than the total net harm to the Y-people by the occurrence of Y.

Negative Wide Average Person-Affecting View:

> An outcome X is worse for people if the *average net harm per person* to the X-people by the occurrence of X would be greater than the average net harm per person to the Y-people by the occurrence of Y.

On both these views, B is worse than A. That is to say, both views would say that the harm to the 2-people would be justified by the harm-reducing effect that the presence of these people has on (many of) the 1-people.

Of the two views, the average view is the less plausible one. Adding extra lives does not increase the average harm per person if the quality of life of the new people is the same or better than those who preceded them. Thus twelve billion poor quality lives is no

---

[45] Parfit, Derek, *Reasons and Persons*. (emphasis added).
[46] Ibid. (emphasis added).

worse, on the average view, than six billion lives of the same quality. But it surely must be worse to inflict that same harm on double the number of people. The total view can avoid this problem. The total harm in a world with twelve billion poor quality lives is greater than that in a world with six billion lives of the same quality. Thus the negative wide total person-affecting view provides one answer about when extra lives may be created in order to reduce the harm to already existent people. We may do so when we thereby minimize the total harm that people suffer.

Some may find this answer unsatisfactory on the grounds that it is concerned only with how much harm there is and not at all with how that harm is distributed and how it is brought about. For example, some may think that it makes a difference whether a larger number of people are each suffering lesser harm or whether a smaller number of people are each suffering greater harm. On this view, it may be worse to create fewer people who suffer more than it would be to create more people who suffer less, even if the total amounts of harm are equivalent. Others may think that it is at least somewhat worse to bring about harm by causing people to exist than it is to allow harm to result from failing to bring people into existence. This may be because they think that actively bringing about harm is worse than passively doing so. More plausibly it may be because they think that creating new people, and thereby harming them, in order to make our own lives less bad, is to treat those new people as mere means to our ends. On this view, there may be a presumption against creating people in order to make our lives go less well. Although that presumption may be defeated where the reduction in harm is sufficiently great, the harm of creating people cannot be justified by merely an equivalent reduction in the harm to already existing people.

Some people may be surprised that a person-affecting view can be subjected to criticisms—about distribution of harm, for example—that are typically levelled at (impersonal) utilitarian views. However, both the wide total person-affecting view and the wide average person-affecting view may, in fact, not be person-affecting at all. Derek Parfit recognizes this when he says that each of the two wide person-affecting views 'restates the impersonal principle in person-affecting form'[47] or 'person-affecting terms'.[48] It is far from clear whether the principles are person-affecting *at all* if they are actually impersonal principles in disguise. An impersonal view does not become a person-affecting one simply because it is stated in a way that sounds person-affecting. Impersonal principles are not concerned with the impact an action has on particular people but are rather concerned with the impact an action has on people in general. It is unsurprising, therefore, that such views will not be able to account adequately for concerns about the harm done to particular people by being brought into existence.

This is not to say that every possible wide person-affecting principle must succumb to this problem. Perhaps there is a version of this principle that is genuinely person-affecting. In other words, perhaps there is a way of filling out 'less good for the X-people than . . .for the Y-people' in a way that takes account of the impact on particular individual people. Averaging and totalling are not the only ways.

Whether or not this is the case, there are some views that can take account of the concerns about how harms are distributed and brought about. For example, a rights or deontological view may say that some harms are so bad that they may not be inflicted even if failing to inflict them causes greater harm to others. On such a view, for example, it would be wrong to remove somebody's healthy kidney involuntarily even though the harm to a potential recipient of not doing the transplant would be greater than the harm to the involuntary donor of doing it. This is because either the donor has a right not to have his kidney involuntarily removed, or others have a duty not to remove it involuntarily. If there is a

---

[47] Parfit, Derek, *Reasons and Persons*. 400.
[48] Ibid. 401.

right not to be brought into existence—a right that has a bearer only when it is breached—then it might be argued that it would be wrong to create new people even if this reduced the harm to currently existing people. Those who are worried about attributing, to non-existent beings, a right not to be brought into existence, may think of this matter instead in terms of duties not to bring people into existence. These would be duties not to inflict the harm that is inflicted by bringing people into existence. On this deontological view, there is a duty not to bring new people into existence—a duty that may not be violated even if doing so would be less than the harm suffered by existent people in the absence of new people. The idea here is that it would be wrong to create people, even if there are fewer of them, to suffer the final-people fate, in order to spare ourselves (even if there are more of us) that same fate.

Where the rights or duties are absolute, it will not matter how much greater the harm to already existent people is. Where the rights are non-absolute, the harms they protect against may not be inflicted merely for an equivalent harm reduction for others but may be inflicted for a significantly greater harm reduction for others. The stronger the non-absolute right, the greater the harm reduction to others must be.

If we combine my anti-natalist arguments with a rights view in order to answer questions about when, if ever, we may cause new people to exist in order to reduce harm to existing people, our answers will not only depend on what view we take of the strength of rights. They will also depend on what view we take about the magnitude of the harm of coming into existence. The greater the harm, the more likely it is to be protected against by a stronger right.

I have examined a range of views and their implications for the following questions:

1. May we ever create new lives in order to improve the quality of existent lives?
2. If so, under what conditions may we do so?

These views and their implications can be summarized as shown in Figure 6.3.

1. (Narrow) Person-Affecting View[49]	Cannot answer the question.	
2. Negative Average View[50]	Incompatible with the anti-natalist argument	
3. Negative Total View[51]	We may create new people where the total amount of harm in doing so is equivalent to, or less than, the harm that would be suffered by existing people if the new people were not created.	
4. Rights/Deontological View	Creating new people cannot be justified by mere reduction in total harm.	**4a. More stringent rights or duty view:** Creating new people can never be justified by any reduction in total harm, no matter how great that reduction may be.
		4b. Less stringent rights or duty view: Creating new people may be justified by substantial (but not mere) reduction in total harm.

Figure 6.3.

[49] I put 'Narrow' in parenthesis, because I have now made it clear that the narrow person-affecting view may be the only truly person-affecting view, although I have indicated that it may still be possible to formulate a wide person-affecting view that is also truly person-affecting.

[50] I refer to this simply as the Negative Average View rather than the Negative Wide Average Person-Affecting view, because we have now seen that the 'person-affecting' label is misleading, and if that is so then the adjective 'wide' is also unnecessary.

[51] I refer to this simply as the Negative Total View rather than the Negative Wide Total Person-Affecting view, because we have now seen that the 'person-affecting' label is misleading, and if that is so then the adjective 'wide' is also unnecessary.

Only the negative total view and the rights or deontological view are plausible candidates for answering anti-natalist questions about when procreation may be permitted in order to prevent further harm to existent people. Although both the negative total view and the less stringent rights or deontological view do permit some creation of new people, they are both compatible with anti-natalism. This is because they only permit the creation of new people as an interim measure as a way of phasing out humanity with the least moral costs. The more stringent rights or deontological view is clearly compatible with anti-natalism.

It is not clear whether the conditions of either the negative total view or the less stringent rights or duty view are met in our world. In other words, it is not obvious that creating new people would reduce total harm at all (to meet the total view's condition) or whether it would reduce it enough (to satisfy the condition of the less stringent rights or duty view). Although phased extinction may very likely reduce the number of people suffering the final-people fate, it may either increase the total harm (because more people are harmed) or not reduce the total harm enough to warrant harming those who are brought into existence. In addition to the obvious normative questions there are also important empirical ones.

Whether or not the conditions of the total view or the less stringent rights or duty view are met, ordinary procreators or potential procreators cannot currently appeal to them to justify their reproducing. This is because the population-related quality of life problems currently faced are those resulting from increasing not decreasing population. And even if the population growth started to taper off or transform into gradual population decline, that would still not be enough. It is only in situations of very rapid population reduction or of reduction back to levels that humans exceeded millennia ago, that questions about creating people to reduce harm could even arise. We are nowhere near there.

EXTINCTION

My arguments in this chapter and previous ones imply that it would be better if humans (and other species) became extinct. All things being equal, my arguments also suggest that it would be better if this occurred sooner rather than later. These conclusions are deeply unsettling to many people. I shall now assess that common response in order to determine whether the prospect of human extinction really is to be regretted, and whether it really would be better for it to occur sooner rather than later.

The human species, like every other species, will eventually become extinct.[52] Many people are disturbed by this prospect and take comfort only in the hope that it may still be a very long time until this occurs.[53] Others are not so sure that our species has a long future. In every generation there are the few who believe that 'the end is nigh'. Often these views are the product of uninformed, often religiously inspired, eschatology, if not of mental disorder. Sometimes, however, they are not.[54] There are those who believe that not only external threats, such as asteroid impact, but also current human practices, including non-sustainable consumption, environmental damage, new and recrudescent diseases, and nuclear or biological weapons, pose a serious threat to the long-term future of humanity. For others, the argument for more imminent extinction is not empirical but

---

[52] As James Lenman says, the 'Second Law of Thermodynamics will get us in the end in the fantastically unlikely event that nothing else does first'. See his 'On Becoming Extinct', *Pacific Philosophical Quarterly*, 83 (2002) 254.

[53] There is the joke about the old lady who attended a lecture on the future of the universe. Afterwards she asked the speaker a question: 'Excuse me, Professor, but when did you say that the universe would come to an end?' 'In about four billion years', replied the speaker. 'Thank God,' remarked the old lady, 'I thought that you said four *million*.'

[54] Rees, Martin, *Our Final Hour: A Scientist's Warning* (New York: Basic Books, 2003).

philosophical. Reasoning probabilistically, they argue that we are destined to 'doom soon'.[55]

I shall not assess arguments and evidence for competing views about when human extinction will occur. We know it will occur, and this fact has a curious effect on my argument. In a strange way it makes my argument an *optimistic* one. Although things are now not the way they should be—there *are* people when there should be none—things will someday be the way they should be—there will be no people. In other words, although things are now bad, they will be better, even if they first get worse with the creation of new people. Some may wish to be spared this kind of optimism, but some optimists may take a measure of comfort in this observation.

Two means of extinction

It would be helpful to distinguish between two ways in which a species can become extinct. The first is for it to be *killed* off. The second is for it to *die* off. We might call the first 'killing-extinction' and the second either 'dying-extinction' or 'non-generative extinction'. When a species is killed off, extinction is brought about by killing members of the species until there are no more of them. This killing may be by humans or it may be by the hand of nature (or by humans forcing the hand of nature). By contrast, when a species dies off, extinction is brought about by a failure to replace those members of the species whose lives come to an inevitable natural end.

It should be clear that the two means of extinction can overlap. What often happens is that so many members of a species are killed off, that the remaining ones cannot effectively replace themselves and those who were killed, and thus when they then die out the species becomes extinct. Alternatively, when a species fails to

[55] Leslie, John, *The End of the World: The Science and Ethics of Human Extinction* (London: Routledge, 1996).

reproduce adequately, the species is brought to extinction by the killing of the few remaining members of the species.

Notwithstanding this overlap, the distinction between the two kinds of extinction (or, if you prefer, the two features of extinction) is helpful. There are clear differences between the two. Most obviously, killing-extinction cuts lives short, whereas dying-extinction does not. Although it may be bad for anyone of us to die, it is still worse to die earlier than we need to. Secondly, there is a moral difference between some cases of killing-extinction and cases of dying-extinction. Were anti-natalists to become pro-mortalists and embark on a 'speciecide' programme of killing humans, their actions would be plagued by moral problems that would not be faced by dying-extinction. Humans killing their own species to extinction is troubling for all the reasons that killing is troubling. It is (usually) bad for those who are killed, and unlike dying (from natural causes), it is a bad that could be avoided (until dying occurs). Although we can regret somebody's death from natural causes at the end of a full life span, we cannot say that any wrong has been done, whereas we *can* say that a moral agent killing somebody, without proper justification, is wrong.

In pointing to both these differences, I assume that death is bad for the one who dies. The view that death is a harm to the one who dies is not an unreasonable view. Indeed it is the common sense view and underlies many important judgements we make. It has been challenged nonetheless. I shall consider this philosophical challenge in the concluding chapter, not in order to defend or reject it, but to show its relevance.

Three concerns about extinction

There are three ways in which extinction might be thought to be bad:

1. Where extinction is brought about by killing, it might be thought to be bad because it cuts lives short.

2. Whichever way extinction is brought about, it might be thought to be bad for those who precede it.
3. The state of extinction might be thought to be bad, in itself. On this view, a world in which there are no people (or other conscious beings) is regrettable in its own right, irrespective of the significance of this state of affairs for earlier beings.[56]

We can make most sense of the first and second bases for regret. Unless people's lives are not worth continuing, cutting their lives short makes their lives still worse—one adds an early death to all the other harms of coming into existence. But extinction need not be brought about this way. Indeed, desisting from creating further people is the best way of ensuring that future people's lives are not cut short. There simply would not be any people whose lives could be cut short.

But this option does not avoid the second concern about extinction. The last generation to die out would bear heavy burdens. First, its hopes and desires for the future beyond itself would be thwarted. Although such hopes and desires of the penultimate and previous generations would also be thwarted, the harm to the final generation would be most severe because its hopes and desires for the future beyond itself would be most radically thwarted. There would be *no* future beyond itself, whereas there would be at least some future beyond the penultimate generation and a little more for each of the earlier generations. The second and more obvious burden for the final generation is that it would live in a world in which the structures of

[56] It is noteworthy that human concern about human extinction takes a different form from human concern (where there is any) about the extinction of non-human species. Most humans who are concerned about the extinction of non-human species are not concerned about the individual animals whose lives are cut short in the passage to extinction, even though that is one of the best reasons to be concerned about extinction (at least in its killing form). The popular concern about animal extinction is usually concern for humans—that we shall live in a world impoverished by the loss of one aspect of faunal diversity, that we shall no longer be able to behold or use that species of animal. In other words, none of the typical concerns about human extinction are applied to non-human species extinction.

society would gradually break down. There would be no younger working generation growing the crops, preserving order, running hospitals and homes for the aged, and burying the dead.

The situation is a bleak one indeed and we can certainly say that looming extinction would be bad for the final people in this way. It is hard to know whether their suffering would be any greater than that of so many people within each generation. I am not at all sure that it would, but let us imagine the opposite for the moment. In order to determine whether this regrettable feature of impending extinction is bad all things considered, we must take account not only of the final people's interests, but also of the harm that is avoided by not producing new generations.

Whenever humanity comes to an end, there will be serious costs for the last people. Either they will be killed or they will languish from the consequences of dwindling population and the collapse of social infrastructure. All things being equal, nothing is gained if this happens later. The same suffering occurs. But there is a cost that does not have to be paid if extinction occurs earlier—the cost to the intervening new generations, those that exist between the present generation and final one. The case for earlier extinction is thus strong.

At best, the production of a limited number of future people, as the discussion in 'Phased Extinction' showed, could be justified as part of a programme of phased extinction, whereby the number of people who will suffer the fate of the final generation is radically reduced from its current billions. However, whether the number of people could be reduced fast enough without the costs of rapid population decline, to a level where the number of final people was small enough to offset the harm to intervening generations, is a difficult one to answer. Whatever the answer, we can say that extinction within a few generations is to be preferred to extinction only after innumerably more generations. Earlier extinction may be worse for some people, but it does not follow that it is worse all things considered.

Whether extinction occurs earlier or later, the third concern is relevant. This is the concern that a world without humans is bad in itself—it is incomplete or deficient. Widespread though this concern is, it is very difficult to make sense of it if one accepts, as most people do, the asymmetry of pain and pleasure. A world without any humans (or other conscious beings) cannot be bad for those who would have existed had extinction not occurred. Indeed, as I have argued, the alternative scenario in which they would have been brought into existence would have been bad for them. A world devoid of such beings is, in this way, a better world. There is no harm in such a world.

Now it might be objected that although a world without humans is better for those humans who would otherwise have existed, a world without humans would be worse in other ways. For example, it would lack moral agents and rational deliberators, and it would be somewhat less diverse. There are a number of problems with such arguments. First, what is so special about a world that contains moral agents and rational deliberators? That humans value a world that contains beings such as themselves says more about their inappropriate sense of self-importance than it does about the world. (Is the world intrinsically better for having six-legged animals? And if so, why? Would it be better still if there were also seven-legged animals?) Although humans may value moral agency and rational deliberation, it is far from clear that these features of our world have value *sub specie aeternitatis*. Thus if there were no more humans there would also be nobody to regret that state of affairs. Nor is it clear why a less diverse world is worse if there is nobody deprived of that diversity.[57] Finally, even if we think that such factors as moral agency, rationality, and diversity enhance the world, it is highly implausible that their value

[57] Although earlier people might regret the prospect of these later states of affairs, we are now examining the third (and not the second) of the three concerns about extinction, whereby the state of extinction is bad independently of the interests of those who precede it.

outweighs the vast amount of suffering that comes with human life. It strikes me, therefore, that the concern that humans will not exist at some future time is either a symptom of the human arrogance that our presence makes the world a better place or is some misplaced sentimentalism.

Many people mourn the prospect of human extinction. Were this extinction both imminent and known to be so, distress about the end of humanity would become much more acute. That distress and sadness, however, would be but another feature of the suffering that foreshadowed the end of human life.

7

Conclusion

So I have praised the dead that are already dead more than the living that are yet alive; but better than both of them is he who has not yet been, who has not seen the evil work that is done under the sun.

Ecclesiastes 1:2–4

There was a young man of Cape Horn
Who wished that he had never been born;
And he wouldn't have been
If his father had seen
That the tip of the rubber was torn.

Unknown[1]

---

[1] I am grateful to Tony Holiday for first drawing this limerick to my attention. Arthur Deex, expert on limericks, kindly gave me some of the history of this one. The version here is evidently a naughty spoof, by an unknown author, of Edward Lear's original:

> There was an Old Man of Cape Horn,
> Who wished he had never been born;
> So he sat on a chair
> Till he died of despair
> That dolorous Man of Cape Horn.

(Jackson, Holbrook, (ed.) *The Complete Nonsense of Edward Lear* (London: Faber & Faber, 1948) 51.) For other variants see Legman, G. *The Limerick: 1700 Examples with Notes, Variants and Index* (New York: Bell Publishing Company, 1969) 188, 425.

COUNTERING
THE COUNTER-INTUITIVENESS
OBJECTION

The view that coming into existence is always a harm runs counter to most people's intuitions. They think that this view simply cannot be right. Its implications, discussed in Chapters 4 to 6, do not fare any better in the court of common intuitions. The idea that people should not have babies, that there is a presumption in favour of abortion (at least in the earlier stages of gestation), and that it would be best if there were no more conscious life on the planet is likely to be dismissed as ridiculous. Indeed, some people are likely to find these views deeply offensive.

A number of philosophers have rejected other views because they imply that it would be better not to bring new people into existence. We already saw, in the previous chapter, that a number of thinkers reject the maximin principle because it implies that there should be no more people. There are other examples, however. Peter Singer rejects a 'moral ledger' view of utilitarianism, whereby the creation of an unsatisfied preference is a kind of 'debit' that is cancelled only when that preference is satisfied. He says that his view must be rejected because it entails that it would be wrong 'to bring into existence a child who will on the whole be very happy, and will be able to satisfy nearly all her preferences, but will still have some preferences unsatisfied'.[2] Nils Holtug rejects frustrationism[3] — the view that while the frustration of preferences has negative value, the satisfaction of preferences simply avoids negative value and contributes nothing positive. Frustrationism implies that we harm people by bringing them into existence if they will have frustrated desires (which everybody

[2] Singer, Peter, *Practical Ethics*, 2nd edn. (Cambridge: Cambridge University Press, 1993) 129.
[3] This view, also known as anti-frustrationism, was discussed in the penultimate section ('Other asymmetries') of Chapter 2.

has). Thus he dismisses frustrationism as 'implausible, indeed deeply counter-intuitive'.[4] Of the implication that it is 'wrong to have a child whose life is much better than the life of anyone we know', he says: 'Surely, this cannot be right.'[5]

I now turn to the question whether it matters that my conclusions are so counter-intuitive. Are my arguments instances of reason gone mad? Should my conclusions be dismissed on account of being so eccentric? Although I understand what motivates these questions, my answer to each of them is an emphatic 'no'.

At the outset, it is noteworthy that a view's counter-intuitiveness cannot by itself constitute a decisive consideration against it. This is because intuitions are often profoundly unreliable—a product of mere prejudice. Views that are taken to be deeply counter-intuitive in one place and time are often taken to be obviously true in another. The view that slavery is wrong, or the view that there is nothing wrong with 'miscegenation', were once thought to be highly implausible and counter-intuitive. They are now taken, at least in many parts of the world, to be self-evident. It is not enough, therefore, to find a view or its implications counter-intuitive, or even offensive. One has to examine the arguments for the disliked conclusion. Most of those who have rejected the view that it is wrong to create more people have done so without assessing the argument for that conclusion. They have simply assumed that this view must be false.

One reason against making this assumption is that the conclusion follows from views that are not only accepted by most people but are also quite reasonable. As I explained in Chapter 2, the asymmetry of pleasure and pain constitutes the best explanation of a number of important moral judgements about creating new people. All my argument does is uncover that asymmetry and to show where it leads.

[4] Holtug, Nils, 'On the value of coming into existence', *The Journal of Ethics*, 5 (2001) 383.
[5] Ibid.

It might be suggested, however, that my argument should be understood as a *reductio ad absurdum* of the commitment to asymmetry. In other words, it might be said that accepting my conclusion is more counter-intuitive than rejecting asymmetry. Thus, if one is faced with the choice between accepting my conclusion and rejecting asymmetry, the latter is preferable.

There are a number of problems with this line of argument. First, we should remember just what it is to which we are committed if we reject asymmetry. Of course, there are various ways of rejecting asymmetry, but the least implausible way would be by denying that absent pleasures are 'not bad' and claiming instead that they are 'bad'. This would commit us to saying that we *do* have a (strong?) moral reason and thus a presumptive duty, based on the interests of future possible happy people, to create those people. It would also commit us to saying that we can create a child for that child's sake and that we should regret, for the sake of those happy people whom we could have created but did not create, that we did not create them. Finally, it would commit us not only to regretting that parts of the earth and all the rest of the universe are uninhabited, but also to regretting this out of concern for those who could otherwise have come into existence in these places.

Matters become still worse if we attempt to abandon asymmetry in another way—by claming that absent pains in Scenario B are merely 'not bad'. That would commit us to saying that we have no moral reason, grounded in the interests of a possible future suffering person, to avoid creating that person. We could no longer regret, based on the interests of a suffering child, that we created that child. Nor could we regret, for the sake of miserable people suffering in some part of the world, that they were ever created.

Those who treat my argument as a *reductio* of asymmetry may find it easier to *say* that they are prepared to abandon asymmetry than actually to *embrace* the implications of doing so. It certainly will not suffice to say that it is better to give up asymmetry and then to proceed, in their ethical theorizing and in their practice, as though asymmetry still held. At the very least, then, my argument should force them to wrestle with the full implications of rejecting asymmetry, which extend well beyond those that I have outlined. I doubt very much that many of those who say that they would rather give up asymmetry really would abandon it.

A second problem with treating my argument as a *reductio* of asymmetry is that although my conclusions may be counter-intuitive, the dominant intuitions in this matter seem thoroughly untrustworthy. This is so for two reasons.

First, why should we think that it is acceptable to cause great harm to somebody—which the arguments in Chapter 3 show we do whenever we create a child—when we could avoid doing so without depriving that person of anything? In other words, how reliable can an intuition be if, even absent the interests of others, it allows the infliction of great harm that could have been avoided without *any* cost to the person who is harmed? Such an intuition would not be worthy of respect in any other context. Why should it be thought to have such force only in procreative contexts?

Secondly, we have excellent reason for thinking that pro-natal intuitions are the product of (at least non-rational, but possibly irrational) psychological forces. As I showed in Chapter 3, there are pervasive and powerful features of human psychology that lead people to think that their lives are better than they really are. Thus their judgements are unreliable. Moreover, there is a good evolutionary explanation for the deep-seated belief that people do not harm their children seriously by bringing them into exist-ence. Those who do not have this belief are less likely to repro-duce. Those with reproduction-enhancing beliefs are more likely to breed and pass on whatever attributes incline one to such beliefs.

What is important to both of these reasons is that it is not merely my extreme claim—that coming into existence is a harm even when a life contains only an iota of suffering—that is counter-intuitive. My more moderate claim—that there is sufficient bad in all actual lives to make coming into existence a harm, even if lives with only an iota of bad would not be harmful—is also counter-intuitive. If only the extreme claim ran counter to common intuitions, then these intuitions would be (somewhat) less suspect. However, then it would have to be said that my extreme claim would be more palatable if all actual lives were largely devoid of bad. This is because the claim would be primarily of theoretical interest and would have little application for procreation, given that the interests of existent people could more plausibly be thought to outweigh the harm to new people. But it is not merely my extreme claim that runs counter to most people's intuitions. Most people think it is implausible that it is harmful and wrong to start lives filled with as much bad as all actual lives contain. Worse still, those who would treat my argument as a *reductio* of asymmetry should note that their argument could also be used by a species doomed to lives much worse than our own. Although we might see their lives as great harms, if they were subject to the kinds of optimistic psychological forces characteristic of humans they too would argue that it is counter-intuitive to claim that they were harmed by being brought into existence. That which would not be counter-intuitive from our perspective would be counter-intuitive from theirs. Yet we can see, with the benefit of some distance from their lives, that little store should be placed on their intuitions about this matter. Something similar can be said about the common human intuition that creating (most) humans is not a harm.[6]

---

[6] As it happens, not all humans share the common intuition that procreation is morally acceptable. There are a non-negligible number of reasonable people who accept an anti-natal view. Not infrequently we hear of people who say that ours is not the sort of world into which children should be brought. The underlying idea is that we live in a world of suffering—a claim I defended in the final section of Chapter 3—and it would be best to avoid creating any new victims of such suffering. I am ready to admit that there are relatively few people who think this, and fewer still who have the strength to act on it, but they are not a lunatic fringe. Moreover, others can understand and make sense of their views and motivations,

There are good reasons, then, for *not* treating my conclusion as a *reductio* of asymmetry. In short, when one has a powerful argument, based on highly plausible premises, for a conclusion that if acted upon would reduce suffering without depriving the suffering person of anything, but which is rejected merely because of primal psychological features that compromise our judgement, then the counter-intuitiveness of the conclusion should not count against it. No doubt there will be some people who are unconvinced by this. If the reason for this is that they take the (alleged) absurdity of my conclusion as axiomatic, then there is nothing that I could say that would convince them. Whatever argument I mustered for my conclusion they would consider refuted by the conclusion it generated. This, however, would not demonstrate a defect in my argument. It would demonstrate only that the negation of my conclusion had attained the status of dogma. There is nothing one can say to convince the dogmatic.

There are some people, and I am among them, who think that there is nothing implausible either in the view that coming into existence is always a harm or in the view that we ought not to have children.[7] It is highly unlikely that a large proportion of humanity

even if they do not agree or follow suit. I agree that the suffering that potential people are likely to endure is sufficient for it to be preferable that they not come into existence. My argument in Chapter 2 extends this widely intelligible intuition and shows that even much less suffering—indeed any suffering at all—would be sufficient to make coming into existence a harm. I emphasize again that although my argument suggests that so long as there is anything bad in a life it is better not to start it, if the amount of bad in a life were truly miniscule then it need not be wrong to have children. This is because the harm could more plausibly be outweighed by the benefits to others. However, as I argued in Chapter 3, the harm in every life is far from miniscule. People's lives, even the most blessed ones, go much worse than is usually thought. Moreover, there is little reason for anybody to think that a potential child will be among the most blessed. There are simply too many things that can go wrong.

[7] Among philosophers, these include not only Christoph Fehige and Seana Shiffrin, both of whom were discussed in the penultimate section of Chapter 2, but also Hermann Vetter, 'Utilitarianism and New Generations', *Mind*, 80/318 (1971) 301–2.

will come to share this view. That is deeply regrettable—because of the immense amount of suffering that this will cause between now and the ultimate demise of humanity.

RESPONDING TO THE OPTIMIST

By most accounts, the views I have defended in this book are rather pessimistic. Pessimism, like optimism, can mean different things, of course.[8] One kind of pessimism or optimism is about the facts. Here pessimists and optimists disagree about what is or will be the case. Thus, they might disagree about whether there is more pleasure or pain in the world at any given time or about whether some person will or will not recover from cancer. A second kind of pessimism and optimism is not about the facts, but about an evaluation of the facts. Here pessimists and optimists disagree not about what is or will be the case, but instead about whether what is or will be the case is good or bad. An optimist of this kind might agree with the pessimist, for example, that there is more pain than pleasure, but think that the pain is worth the pleasure. Alternatively, the pessimist might agree with the optimist that there is more pleasure than pain, but deny that even that quantity of pleasure is worth the pain. The 'is or will be' clause in both the factual and evaluative versions refers to a third distinction, but one that obviously cuts across the first two. Very often pessimism and optimism are understood to be future-oriented—to refer to assessments of how things will be. However, both terms are also sometimes used in either a non-future-oriented or alternatively a timeless sense.

The view that coming into existence is always a serious harm is pessimistic in both a factual and evaluative sense. I have suggested, factually, that human life contains much more pain (and other

---

[8] Much of the rest of this paragraph is drawn from my Introduction to David Benatar (ed.), *Life, Death and Meaning* (Lanham MD: Rowman & Littlefield, 2004) 15.

negative things) than people realize. Evaluatively, I have endorsed the asymmetry of pleasure and pain and suggested that whereas life's pleasures do not make life worth starting, life's pains do make life not worth starting. In future-oriented terms, my view is pessimistic in most ways but could be construed as optimistic in one way. Given how much suffering occurs every minute, there is very good reason to think that there will be much more suffering before sentient life comes to an end, although I cannot predict with any certainty just *how* much more suffering there will be. All things being equal, the longer sentient life continues, the more suffering there will be. However, there is an optimistic spin on my view, as I noted in Chapter 6. Humanity and other sentient life will eventually come to an end. For those who judge the demise of humanity to be a bad thing, the prediction that this is what will occur is a pessimistic one. By contrast, combining my evaluation that it would be better if there where no more people with the prediction that there will come a time when there will be no more people yields an optimistic assessment. Things are bad now, but they will not always be bad. On the other hand, again, if one thinks that the better state of affairs will be a long time in coming, then one could characterize the view that it is far off as pessimistic.

Pessimism tends not to be well received. On account of the psychological dispositions to think that things are better than they are, which I discussed in Chapter 3, people want to hear positive messages. They want to hear that things are better than they think, not worse. Indeed, where there is not a pathologizing of pessimism by placing it under the rubric of 'depression', there is often an impatience with or condemnation of it. Some people will have these reactions to the view that coming into existence is always a harm. These optimists will dismiss this view as weak and self-indulgent. They may tell us that we cannot 'cry over spilled milk'. We have already come into existence and there is no use bemoaning that fact in lugubrious self-pitying. We must 'count our blessings', 'make the most of life', 'take pleasure', and 'look on the bright side'.

There are good reasons not to be intimidated by the optimist's chidings. First, optimism cannot be the right view merely because it is cheery, just as pessimism cannot be the right view merely because it is grim. Which view we adopt must depend on the evidence. I have argued in this book that a grim view about coming into existence is the right one.

Secondly, one can regret one's existence without being self-pitying. This is not to say that there is anything wrong with a modicum of self-pity. If one pities others, why should one not pity oneself, at least in moderation? In any event, the view I have defended is not only self-regarding but also other-regarding in its relevance. It provides a basis not only for regretting one's own existence but also for not having children. In other words, it has relevance for milk that has not yet been spilled and need not ever be spilled.

Thirdly, there is nothing in my view that suggests we should not 'count our blessings' if by this one means that one should be pleased that one's life is not still worse than it is. A few of us are very lucky *relative* to much of the species. There is no harm—and there may be benefits—in recognizing this. But the injunction to count one's blessings is much less compelling when it entails deceiving oneself into thinking that one was actually lucky to have come into existence. It is like being grateful that one is in a first-class cabin on the *Titanic* as one awaits descent to one's watery grave. It may be better to die in first-class than in steerage, but not so much better as to count oneself very lucky. Nor does my view preclude our making the most of life or taking pleasure whenever we can (within the constraints of morality). I have argued that our lives are very bad. There is no reason why we should not try to make them less so, on condition that we do not spread the suffering (including the harm of existence).

Finally, the optimist's impatience with or condemnation of pessimism often has a smug macho tone to it (although males have no monopoly of it). There is a scorn for the perceived weakness of the pessimist who should instead 'grin and bear it'. This view is defective for the same reason that macho views about other kinds of suffering are defective. It is an indifference to or inappropriate denial of suffering, whether one's own or that of others. The injunction to 'look on the bright side' should be greeted with a large dose of both scepticism and cynicism. To insist that the bright side is always the right side is to put ideology before the evidence. Every cloud, to change metaphors, may have a silver lining, but it may very often be the cloud rather than the lining on which one should focus if one is to avoid being drenched by self-deception. Cheery optimists have a much less realistic view of themselves than do those who are depressed.[9]

Optimists might respond that even if I am right that coming into existence is always a harm it is better not to dwell on this fact, for to dwell on it only compounds the harm by making one miserable. There is an element of truth here. However, we need to put it in perspective. An acute sense of regret about one's own existence is probably the most effective way to avoid inflicting that same harm on others. If people are able to recognize the harm of having come into existence but still remain cheery without slipping into the practice of making new people, their cheer should not be begrudged. However, if their cheer comes at the cost of self-deception and resultant procreation, then they are susceptible to a charge of having lost perspective. They may be happier than others, but that does not make them right.

DEATH AND SUICIDE

Many people believe that it is an implication of the view that coming into existence is always a harm that it would be preferable to

[9] For a discussion of this see Taylor, Shelley E., and Brown, Jonathon D., 'Illusion and Well-Being: A Social Psychological Perspective on Mental Health', *Psychological Bulletin*, 103/2 (1998) 193–210.

die than to continue living. Some people go so far as to say that the view that coming into existence is a harm implies the desirability not simply of death but of suicide.

There is nothing incoherent about the view that coming into existence is a harm and that if one does come into existence ceasing to exist is better than continuing to exist. This is the view expressed in the following quotation from Sophocles:

> Never to have been born is best
> But if we must see the light, the next best
> Is quickly returning whence we came.
> When youth departs, with all its follies,
> Who does not stagger under evils? Who escapes them?[10]

And it is implicit in, or at least compatible with, Montesquieu's claim that 'Men should be bewailed at their birth and not at their death'.[11]

Nevertheless, the view that coming into existence is always a harm does *not imply* that death is better than continuing to exist, and a fortiori that suicide is (always) desirable.[12] Life may be sufficiently bad that it is better not to come into existence, but not so bad that it is better to cease existing. It will be recalled, from Chapter 2, that it is possible to have different evaluations of future-life and present-life cases. I explained in that chapter

---

[10] Sophocles, *Oedipus at Colonus*, lines 1224–31.

[11] Montesquieu, 'Letter Forty', *Persian Letters,* trans. John Davidson, 1 (London: Gibbings & Company, 1899) 123.

[12] Commenting on the apparent oddity of regretting one's existence yet clinging to life, Woody Allen speaks of two Jews eating in a restaurant in the Catskills. The one says to the other: 'The food here is terrible.' The other replies: 'Yes, and the portions are so small.' At one level, there is nothing strange about disliking some food and complaining that there is not more of it. Not having enough food—going hungry—is bad even if the alternative is to satiate oneself with food that does not taste very nice. The reason why the Woody Allen image is odd and funny is that we assume that the pair are not in need of the extra food—either that their eating is more recreational or that the portions are big *enough*. The same dialogue between two Jews in Auschwitz would not be funny at all, because it wouldn't be odd at all to complain both about the quality and quantity of the food.

that there is good reason for setting the quality threshold for a life worth starting higher than the quality threshold for a life worth continuing. This is because the existent can have interests in continuing to exist, and thus harms that make life not worth continuing must be sufficiently severe to defeat those interests. By contrast, the non-existent have no interest in coming into existence. Therefore, the avoidance of even lesser harms—or, on my view, *any* harm—will be decisive.

Thus, it is because we (usually) have an interest in continuing to exist that death may be thought of as a harm, even though coming into existence is also a harm. Indeed, the harm of death may partially explain why coming into existence is a harm. Coming into existence is bad in part because it invariably leads to the harm of ceasing to exist. That may be behind George Santayana's claim that the 'fact of having been born is a very bad augury for immortality'.[13] That we are born destined to die is, on this view, a great harm.

The view that one has an interest in continuing to live (so long as the quality of one's life has not fallen beneath the lower threshold of a life worth continuing) is a common one. However, it has been subjected to ancient and resilient objections. Epicurus famously argued that death is not bad for the one who dies because so long as one exists, one is not dead, and once death arrives one no longer exists. Thus, my being dead (in contrast to my dying) is not something that I can experience. Nor is it a condition in which I can be. Instead it is a condition in which I am not. Accordingly my death is not something that can be bad for me. Lucretius, a disciple of Epicurus' and thus also an Epicurean, advanced a further argument against death's being a harm. He argued that since we do not regret the period of non-existence before we came into being, we should not regret the non-existence that follows our lives.

[13] Santayana, George, *Reason in Religion* (vol. iii of *The Life of Reason*) (New York: Charles Scribner's Sons, 1922) 240.

The Epicurean arguments assume that death is the irreversible cessation of existence. Those who think that there is life after death reject this assumption. Whether or not death is bad on this alternative view depends on how good the post-mortem life is. Although this is a topic about which there is much speculation, nothing vaguely testable can be said about it. In considering whether my argument entails that death is preferable to continued life, I shall join the Epicureans in assuming that death is the irreversible cessation of existence.

The view that death is not bad for the one who died is at odds with a number of deeply held views. Among these is the view that murder harms the victim. It is also incompatible with the view that a longer life is, all things being equal, better than a shorter one. And it is in conflict with the view that we ought to respect the wishes of those who are now dead (quite independently of the effect that not doing so would have on the still living). This is because if death is not a harm, then nothing that happens after death can be a harm.

Counter-intuitiveness, by itself, is not enough to show that a view is mistaken, as I have argued. However, there are some important differences between the counter-intuitiveness of the Epicurean arguments and the counter-intuitiveness of my anti-natalist arguments. First, the Epicurean conclusion is more radically counter-intuitive than my conclusion. I suspect that more people think, and feel more strongly, that murder harms the victim than who think that coming into existence is not a harm. Indeed there are very many people who believe that coming into existence is often a harm and there are still more people who believe that it is never a benefit even if they think that it is not also a harm. Yet there are very few people who truly believe that murder does not harm the victim. Even where the victim's life was of a poor quality, it is widely thought that killing that person without his consent (where consent could have been obtained) is to wrong him. Secondly, a precautionary principle applies asymmetrically to the two views. If the Epicurean is wrong, then people's acting on the Epicurean argument (by killing others or themselves) would seriously harm those who were killed. By contrast, if my view is mistaken, people's acting on my view (by having failed to procreate) would not harm those who were not brought into existence. These differences in the counter-intuitiveness of the Epicurean and anti-natal views are not sufficient, however, to dismiss the Epicurean arguments out of hand. Therefore, I turn now to consider, albeit only briefly, responses to both Epicurean arguments.

I start with Lucretius' argument. The best way to respond to this argument is to deny that there is symmetry between pre-vital and post-mortem non-existence.[14] Whereas any one of us could live longer, none of us could have come into existence much earlier. This argument becomes very powerful when we recognize the kind of existence that we value. It is not some 'metaphysical essence', but rather a thicker, richer conception of the self,[15] that embodies one's particular memories, beliefs, commitments, desires, aspirations, and so on. One's identity, in this thicker sense, is constructed from one's particular history. But even if one's metaphysical essence could have come into existence earlier, the history of that being would have been so different that it would not be the same person as one is. Yet, things are quite different at the other end of life. Personal histories—biographies—can be lengthened by not dying sooner. Once one is, one can continue to be for longer. But an earlier coming into existence would have been the coming into existence of a different person—one with whom one might have very little in common.

The most common response to Epicurus' argument is to say that death is bad for the person who dies because it deprives that person of future life and the positive features thereof. The deprivation account of death's badness does not entail that death is *always* bad

[14] The term 'pre-vital non-existence' is Frederik Kaufman's. See his 'Pre-Vital and Post-Mortem Non-Existence', *American Philosophical Quarterly*, 36/1 (1999) 1–19.
[15] The argument I outline here is Frederik Kaufman's. See his 'Pre-Vital and Post-Mortem Non-Existence'.

for the one who dies. Indeed, where the further life of which some-body is deprived is of a sufficiently poor quality, death is not bad for that person. Instead it is good. The Epicurean argument, however, is that death is *never* bad for the person who dies. The deprivation account is a response to this, and claims that death can *sometimes* be bad for the person who dies. On the deprivation account, even though a person no longer exists after his death, it is still true that his death deprives him, the 'ante-mortem'[16] person, of the further life he could have enjoyed.

Defenders of Epicurus take issue with the deprivation account. One objection is that advocates of the deprivation account cannot say *when* the harm of death occurs—that is, they cannot date the time of the harm. The time of the harm cannot be when death oc-curs because by that time the person who non-Epicureans say is harmed by the death no longer exists. And if it is the ante-mortem person who is harmed, one cannot say that the time at which that person is harmed is the time of his death, because that would in-volve backward causation—a later event causing an earlier harm. One response to this challenge is to say that the time at which death harms is 'always' or 'eternally'.[17] George Pitcher offers a helpful analogy. He says that if 'the world should be blasted to smithereens during the next presidency. . .this would make it true (be respons-ible for the fact) that even now, during. . .[the current president's] term, he is the penultimate president of the United States'.[18] Simil-arly, one's later death makes it true that even now one is doomed not to live longer than one will. Just as there is no backward caus-ation in the case of the penultimate president, so there is no back-ward causation in a death that harms one all along.

---

[16] The term 'ante-mortem' person is George Pitcher's. See his 'The Misfortunes of the Dead', *American Philosophical Quarterly*, 21/2 (1984) 183–8.

[17] The term 'eternally' is Fred Feldman's, See his 'Some Puzzles About the Evil of Death', *Philosophical Review*, 100/2 (1991) 205–27.

[18] Pitcher, George, 'The Misfortunes of the Dead', 188.

There is a more fundamental (but not clearly more powerful) objection to the deprivation account. Defenders of Epicurus simply deny that those who have ceased to exist can be deprived of anything. David Suits, for example, argues that although the ante-mortem person may indeed be worse off than he would otherwise have been had he lived longer, being worse off in this 'purely relational' way is not thought to be sufficient to show that he is harmed.[19] He argues further that even if it were, there cannot be real deprivation if there is nobody *left* to be deprived. One can only be deprived if one exists.

But here we seem to have an impasse. Defenders of the deprivation account seem to think that death is different and that it is the one kind of case in which somebody can be deprived without existing. Epicureans, by contrast, insist that death cannot be different and we must treat deprivation in the same way here as we do in all other cases. In no other cases can a person be deprived without existing, so a person cannot be deprived by death, given that death brings the end of his existence.

Perhaps there is a way to get past this impasse, but I shall not seek it now. I have shown that the view that coming into existence is a harm does not *entail* the view that ceasing to exist is better than continuing to exist. One can maintain that both are harms. Epicureans deny that ceasing to exist can be a harm. They may also be committed to saying that death can never be *good* for the one who dies, no matter how bad that person's life has become. Following the Epicurean reasoning, death can never benefit a person because so long as he is, death is not, and when death arrives he no longer is. Death cannot *spare* anybody from anything any more than it can *deprive* anybody of anything.

[19] Suits, David B., 'Why death is not bad for the one who died', *American Philosophical Quarterly*, 38/1 (2001) 69–84.

Those who reject the Epicurean view can hold one of a number of positions:

a) Death is always a harm.
b) Death is always a benefit.
c) Death is sometimes a harm and sometimes a benefit.

The first option is implausible. Life can be so bad that it is better to die. Those who deny that coming into existence is always a harm, obviously reject the second option. On this view, coming into existence is not bad and may even be good, and continuing to exist is good so long as the quality of one's life is of a sufficiently high standard. Thus death cannot always be a benefit. I said earlier that those who adopt the view that coming into existence is always a harm can also reject the second option. They can argue that whereas we have no interest in coming into existence, once we do exist, we have an interest in continuing to exist. On the assumption that this interest is not always defeated by the poor quality of life, death is not always a benefit. But is this assumption reasonable, given how serious a harm I have said it is to come into existence? I think that it is, but saying that it is a reasonable assumption is not to make a very strong claim. It is to say only that the quality of life is not *always* so poor that ceasing to exist is a benefit. It leaves wide open the question of how often it is not so poor.

This is not a question I need to answer. By a principle of autonomy we parcel out the authority to make decisions about the quality of individual lives to those whose lives they are. Unlike autonomous decisions to procreate, autonomous decisions to continue living or to die are made by those whose lives are in question. It is true that if people's lives are worse than they think (as I argued in Chapter 3) their assessments about whether their lives are worth continuing may be mistaken. Nevertheless, that is the sort of mistake we should allow people to make. It is a mistake, the consequences of which they must bear—unlike the mistake of thinking that the lives of one's potential offspring will be better than one thinks. Similarly, the desire to continue living may or may not be irrational, but even if it is, this is the kind of irrationality, unlike a preference for having come into existence, that should be decisive (at least in practice if not in theory).

Matters are a little different when the decision to end a life is not made by an autonomous being for himself, but is instead made on behalf of a being that lacks the ability to make the judgement for itself (and has left neither an advance directive nor a durable power of attorney). These are the hardest cases. Unlike deciding whether to create a new life, where one can err on the side of caution by not creating a new life, there is no clear side of caution on which to err when it comes to ending a life.

Thus I share a version of the third option listed above—that death is sometimes a harm and sometimes a benefit. This third option is the common sense view, but my version will deviate from the usual interpretation of it. That is to say, it is likely that my version allows for death to be a benefit more often than the usual view. For example, my view would be more tolerant of rational suicide than would the common view. Indeed, I would claim more suicides to be rational than would the common view. In many cultures (including most western cultures), there is immense prejudice against suicide. It is often viewed as cowardly[20] where it is not dismissed as a consequence of mental illness. My view allows the possibility that suicide may more often be rational and may even be more rational than continuing to exist. This is because it may be an irrational love for life that keeps many people alive when their lives have actually become so bad that ceasing to exist would be better. This is the view expressed by the old woman in Voltaire's *Candide*:

A hundred times I wished to kill myself, but my love of life persisted. This ridiculous weakness is perhaps one of the most fatal of our faults.

[20] In other cultures, interestingly, it is the failure to commit suicide in certain circumstances that is viewed as being cowardly.

For what could be more stupid than to go on carrying a burden that we always long to lay down? To loathe, and yet cling to, existence? In short, to cherish the serpent that devours us, until it has eaten our hearts?[21]

This is not to offer a general recommendation of suicide. Suicide, like death from other causes, makes the lives of those who are bereaved much worse. Rushing into one's own suicide can have profound negative impact on the lives of those close to one. Although an Epicurean may be committed to not caring about what happens after his death, it is still the case that the bereaved suffer a harm even if the deceased does not. That suicide harms those who are thereby bereaved is part of the tragedy of coming into existence. We find ourselves in a kind of trap. We have already come into existence. To end our existence causes immense pain to those we love and for whom we care. Potential procreators would do well to consider this trap they lay when they produce offspring. It is not the case that one can create new people on the assumption that if they are not pleased to have come into existence they can simply kill themselves. Once somebody has come into existence and attachments with that person have been formed, suicide can cause the kind of pain that makes the pain of childlessness mild by comparison. Somebody contemplating suicide knows (or should know) this. This places an important obstacle in the way of suicide. One's life may be bad, but one must consider what affect ending it would have on one's family and friends. There will be times when life has become so bad that it is unreasonable for the interests of the loved ones in having the person alive to outweigh that person's interests in ceasing to exist. When this is true will depend in part on particular features of the person for whom continued life is a burden. Different people are able to bear different magnitudes of burden. It may even be indecent for family members to expect that person to continue living. On other occasions one's life may be bad but not so bad as to warrant killing oneself and thereby making

[21] Voltaire, *Candide* (London: Penguin Books, 1997) 32–3.

the lives of one's family and friends still much worse than they already are.

RELIGIOUS VIEWS

There are some people who will reject, on religious grounds, the views that coming into existence is always a harm and that we ought not to have children. For some such people, the Biblical injunction to 'be fruitful and multiply and fill the earth'[22] will constitute a refutation of my views. Such a response assumes, of course, that God exists. This is no place to discuss *God's* existence. Whether or not the (mono-)theists are right, God never came into existence. If they are right, God always existed, and if they are wrong God never existed. Moreover, what I have said about the quality of human (and animal) life would not entail anything about the quality of Divine life. And thus I leave aside the question of God's existence.

The religious response also assumes that Biblical imperatives are the expression of what God requires of us. This may seem uncontroversial for those who accept that the Bible is the word of God. However, very many Biblical commandments are not thought to be binding, even by religious people. For example, no religion I know of currently endorses, as a practical matter, putting to death one's rebellious son, the Biblical commandment to do so notwithstanding.[23] Even the commandment to be fruitful and multiply is not viewed as absolute. For example, Catholicism must exempt priests and nuns from procreation, given that it forbids those occupying such positions from engaging in the intercourse that leads to procreation and prohibits procreation by non-sexual means. Whereas Catholics permit procreation (in the context of marriage) for others, the Shakers advocated celibacy for everybody, including married couples.

[22] Genesis 1:28.   [23] Deuteronomy 21:18–21.

A third and more interesting response to the religious argument is that the religious argument assumes too monolithic a view of religion. Although any one religion is often thought and said to speak with one voice on any given topic, there is in fact a range of divergent views even within a single religion and within a single denomination of a religion. Brief illustration of this can be provided with reference to one's coming into existence.

The epigraphs at the beginning of Chapter 5 show both Jeremiah and Job ruing their births. Job regrets his having been conceived and the fact that he did not die *in utero* or at birth. Jeremiah goes further and curses the man who did not abort him. It is striking how different such views are from those of the cheery fundamentalist with an unsophisticated, monolithic view of the right way. Whereas Jeremiah and Job think and speak freely—even challenge God himself—all too few religious believers follow suit. For them piety precludes such critical thinking and speaking.

Now it might be suggested that both Jeremiah and Job regretted their own existences for reasons specific to the content of their lives—because, for one reason or another, the quality of their lives was poor. On this view, there are some lives of which it is true that it would have been better had they not been started, but it is not true of all lives. That view seems at odds with the epigraph from Ecclesiastes at the beginning of this chapter. Those verses show a Biblical author envying all those who have not come into existence.

Nor is the Bible the only religious text in which we find alternative religious views about the disvalue of coming into existence. The Talmud,[24] for example, briefly records the subject of a fascinating debate between two famous early rabbinic schools—the House of Hillel and the House of Shammai. We are told that they debated the question whether or not it was better for humans to have been created. The House of Hillel, known for its generally more lenient and humane views, maintained that it was indeed

---

[24] Tractate Eruvin 13b.

better that humans were created. The House of Shammai maintained, by contrast, that it would have been better had humans not been created. The Talmud relates that these two schools debated the matter for two and a half years and the issue was eventually settled in favour of the House of Shammai. This is particularly noteworthy, because in cases of disagreement between these two schools, the law almost always follows the House of Hillel. Yet here we have a decision in favour of Shammai, endorsing the view that it would have been better had humans not been created. This kind of second-guessing of God would not cross the minds of the self-consciously pious. But the fact remains that religious traditions can embody views that superficial religious thinkers would take to be antithetical to religiosity. Recognition of this might prevent a quick dismissal of my views on religious grounds.

MISANTHROPY AND PHILANTHROPY

The conclusions I have reached will strike many people as deeply misanthropic. I have argued that life is filled with unpleasantness and suffering, that we should avoid having children, and that it would be best if humanity came to an end sooner rather than later. This may sound like misanthropy. However, the overwhelming thrust of my arguments, as they apply to humans, is philanthropic, not misanthropic. Because my arguments apply not only to humans but also to other sentient animals, my arguments are also zoophilic (in the non-sexual sense of that term). Bringing a sentient life into existence is a harm to the being whose life it is. My arguments suggest that it is wrong to inflict this harm. To argue against the infliction of harm arises from concern for, not dislike of, those who would be harmed. It may seem like an odd kind of philanthropy—one that if acted upon, would lead to the end of all *anthropos*. It is, however, the most effective way of preventing suffering. Not creating a person absolutely guarantees that that potential person will not suffer—because that person will not exist.

Although the arguments I have advanced have not been misanthropic, there is a superb misanthropic argument against having children and in favour of human extinction. This argument rests on the indisputable premiss that humans cause colossal amounts of suffering—both for humans and for non-human animals. In Chapter 3, I provided a brief sketch of the kind of suffering humans inflict on one another. In addition to this, they are the cause of untold suffering to other species. Each year, humans inflict suffering on billions of animals that are reared and killed for food and other commodities or used in scientific research. Then there is the suffering inflicted on those animals whose habitat is destroyed by encroaching humans, the suffering caused to animals by pollution and other environmental degradation, and the gratuitous suffering inflicted out of pure malice.

Although there are many non-human species—especially carnivores—that also cause a lot of suffering, humans have the unfortunate distinction of being the most destructive and harmful species on earth. The amount of suffering in the world could be radically reduced if there were no more humans. Even if the misanthropic argument is not taken to this extreme, it can be used to defend at least a radical reduction of the human population.

Although the end of humanity would greatly reduce the amount of harm, it would not end it all. The remaining sentient beings would continue to suffer and their coming into existence could still be a harm. This is one reason why the misanthropic argument does not go as far as the arguments I have advanced in this book—arguments that arise not from antipathy towards the human species but rather from concern about harms to all sentient beings. Moreover, as resistant as people are to the philanthropic argument, they would be still more resistant to the misanthropic one. But the misanthropic argument is not in the least incompatible with the philanthropic one.

It is unlikely that many people will take to heart the conclusion that coming into existence is always a harm. It is even less likely that many people will stop having children. By contrast, it is quite likely that my views either will be ignored or will be dismissed. As this response will account for a great deal of suffering between now and the demise of humanity, it cannot plausibly be thought of as philanthropic. That is not to say that it is motivated by any malice towards humans, but it does result from a self-deceptive indifference to the harm of coming into existence.

Bibliography

Andrews, Frank M., and Withey, Stephen B., *Social Indicators of Well-Being: Americans' Perspectives of Life Quality* (New York: Plenum Press, 1976).

Bayles, Michael, *Morality and Population Policy* (University of Alabama Press, 1980).

Benatar, David, 'Why it is Better Never to Come into Existence', *American Philosophical Quarterly*, 34/3 (1997) 345–55.

—— 'Cloning and Ethics', *QJMed*, 91 (1998) 165–6.

—— 'The Wrong of Wrongful Life', *American Philosophical Quarterly*, 37/2 (2000) 175–83.

—— 'To Be or Not to Have Been?: Defective Counterfactual Reasoning About One's Own Existence', *International Journal of Applied Philosophy*, 15/2 (2001) 255–66.

—— (ed.) *Life, Death and Meaning* (Lanham MD: Rowman & Littlefield, 2004).

—— 'Sexist Language: Alternatives to the Alternatives', *Public Affairs Quarterly*, 19/1 (2005) 1–9.

—— and Benatar, Michael, 'A Pain in the Fetus: Ending Confusion about Fetal Pain', *Bioethics*, 15/1 (2001) 57–76.

Beyer, Lisa, 'Be Fruitful and Multiply: Criticism of the ultra-Orthodox fashion for large families is coming from inside the community', *Time*, 25 October 1999, 34.

Blackstone, William T., (ed.) *Philosophy and Environmental Crisis* (Athens: University of Georgia Press, 1974) 43–68.

Boonin, David, 'Against the Golden Rule Argument Against Abortion', *Journal of Applied Philosophy*, 14/2 (1997) 187–97.

—— *A Defense of Abortion* (Cambridge: Cambridge University Press, 2003).

Boorse, Christopher, 'On the Distinction between Disease and Illness', *Philosophy and Public Affairs*, 5/1 (1975) 49–68.

Bowring, Philip, 'For Love of Country', *Time*, 11 September 2000, 58.

Breetvelt, I. S., and van Dam, F. S. A. M., 'Underreporting by Cancer Patients: the Case of Response Shift', *Social Science and Medicine*, 32/9 (1991) 981–7.

Brickman, Philip, Coates, Dan, and Janoff-Bulman, Ronnie, 'Lottery Winners and Accident Victims: Is Happiness Relative?', *Journal of Personality and Social Psychology*, 36/8 (1978) 917–27.

Brown, Jonathon D., and Dutton, Keith A., 'Truth and Consequences: the Costs and Benefits of Accurate Self-Knowledge', *Personality and Social Psychology Bulletin*, 21/12 (1995) 1288–96.

Buchanan, Allen, Brock, Dan, Daniels, Norman, and Wikler, Daniel, *From Chance to Choice* (New York: Cambridge University Press, 2000).

Burkett, Elinor, *The Baby Boon: How Family-Friendly America Cheats the Childless*, (New York: The Free Press, 2000).

Cameron, Paul, Titus, Donna G., Kostin, John, and Kostin, Marilyn, 'The Life Satisfaction of Nonnormal Persons', *Journal of Consulting and Clinical Psychology*, 41 (1973) 207–14.

Campbell, Angus, Converse, Philip E., and Rodgers, Willard L., *The Quality of American Life* (New York: Russell Sage Foundation, 1976).

Craig, K. D., Whitfield, M. F., Grunau, R. V., Linton, J., and Hadjistavropoulos, H. D., 'Pain in the Preterm Neonate: Behavioural and Physiological Indices', *Pain*, 52/3 (1993) 287–99.

Diener, Ed., and Diener, Carol, 'Most People are Happy', *Psychological Science*, 7/3 (1996) 181–5.

—— Suh, Eunkook M., Lucas, Richard E., and Smith, Heidi L., 'Subjective Well-Being: Three Decades of Progress', *Psychological Bulletin*, 125/2 (1999) 276–302.

Easterlin, Richard A., 'Explaining Happiness', *Proceedings of the National Academy of Sciences*, 100/19 (2003) 11176–83.

—— 'The Economics of Happiness', *Daedalus*, Spring 2004, 26–33.

Economist, The, 'The incredible shrinking country', *The Economist*, 13 November 2004, 45–6.

Elliot, Robert, 'Regan on the Sorts of Beings that Can Have Rights', *Southern Journal of Philosophy*, 16 (1978) 701–5.

Fehige, Christoph, 'A Pareto Principle for Possible People', in Fehige, Christoph, and Wessels, Ulla, (eds.) *Preferences* (Berlin: Walter de Gruyter, 1998) 508–43.

Feinberg, Joel, 'The Rights of Animals and Unborn Generations', *Rights, Justice and the Bounds of Liberty* (Princeton: Princeton University Press, 1980) 159–84.

—— 'Wrongful Life and the Counterfactual Element in Harming', in *Freedom and Fulfilment* (Princeton: Princeton University Press, 1992) 3–36.

Feldman, Fred, 'Some Puzzles About the Evil of Death', *Philosophical Review*, 100/2 (1991) 205–27.

Flaubert, Gustave, *The Letters of Gustave Flaubert 1830–1857*, trans. Francis Steegmuller (London: Faber & Faber, 1979).

Food and Agriculture Organization of the United Nations, 'Undernourishment Around the World', <http://www.fao/org/DOCREP/005/y7352E/y7352e03.htm> (accessed 14 November 2003).

Freud, Sigmund, *The Standard Edition of the Complete Psychological Works of Sigmund Freud*, vii, trans. James Strachey (London: The Hogarth Press, 1960).

Frey, R. G., 'Rights, Interests, Desires and Beliefs', *American Philosophical Quarterly*, 16/3 (1979) 233–9.

Greenwald, Anthony G., 'The Totalitarian Ego: Fabrication and Revision of Personal History', *American Psychologist*, 35/7 (1980) 603–18.

Griffin, James, *Well-Being* (Oxford: Clarendon Press, 1986).

Hacker, Andrew, 'The Case Against Kids', *The New York Review of Books*, 47/19 (2000) 12–18.

Hare, R. M., 'Abortion and the Golden Rule', *Philosophy and Public Affairs*, 4/3 (1975) 201–22.

—— 'A Kantian Approach to Abortion', *Essays on Bioethics* (Oxford: Clarendon Press, 1993) 168–84.

Haub, Carl, 'How Many People Have Ever Lived on Earth?', <http://www.prb.org/Content/ContentGroups/PTarticle/Oct-Dec02/How_Many_People_Have_Ever_Lived_on_Earth_.htm> (accessed 5 October 2004).

Headey, Bruce, and Wearing, Alexander, 'Personality, Life Events, and Subjective Well-Being: Toward a Dynamic Equilibrium Model', *Journal of Personality and Social Psychology*, 57/4 (1989) 731–9.

Heine, Heinrich, *Morphine*, lines 15–16.

Holtug, Nils, 'On the value of coming into existence', *The Journal of Ethics*, 5 (2001) 361–84.

Hunger Project, The, <http://www.thp.org> (accessed November 2003).

Inglehart, Ronald, *Culture Shift in Advanced Industrial Society* (Princeton: Princeton University Press, 1990).

Jackson, Holbrook, (ed.) *The Complete Nonsense of Edward Lear* (London: Faber & Faber, 1948) 51.

Kagan, Shelly, *The Limits of Morality* (Oxford: Clarendon Press, 1989).

Kates, Carol A., 'Reproductive Liberty and Overpopulation', *Environmental Values*, 13 (2004) 51–79.

Kaufman. Frederik, 'Pre-Vital and Post-Mortem Non-Existence', *American Philosophical Quarterly*, 36/1 (1999) 1–19.

Kavka, Gregory S., 'The Paradox of Future Individuals', *Philosophy and Public Affairs*, 11/2 (1982) 93–112.

Krug, Etienne G., Dahlbeg, Linda L., Mercy, James A., Zwi, Anthony B., and Lozano, Rafael, (eds.) *The World Health Report 2002* (Geneva: WHO, 2002).

Legman, G., *The Limerick: 1700 Examples with Notes, Variants and Index* (New York: Bell Publishing Company, 1969).

Lenman, James, 'On Becoming Extinct', *Pacific Philosophical Quarterly*, 83 (2002) 253–69.

Leslie, John, *The End of the World: The Science and Ethics of Human Extinction* (London: Routledge, 1996).

McGuire, Bill, *A Guide to the End of the World* (New York: Oxford University Press, 2002).

McMahan, Jeff, *The Ethics of Killing: Problems at the Margins of Life* (New York: Oxford University Press, 2002).

McMichael, Anthony, *Human Frontiers, Environments and Disease* (Cambridge: Cambridge University Press, 2001).

Marquis, Don, 'Why Abortion is Immoral', *The Journal of Philosophy*, 86/4 (1989) 183–202.

—— 'Justifying the Rights of Pregnancy: The Interest View', *Criminal Justice Ethics*, 13/1 (1994) 67–81.

Maslow, Abraham, *Motivation and Personality*, 2nd edn. (New York: Harper & Row Publishers, 1970).

Matlin, Margaret W., and Stang, David J., *The Pollyanna Principle: Selectivity in Language, Memory and Thought* (Cambridge MA: Schenkman Publishing Company, 1978).

May, Elaine Tyler, 'Nonmothers as Bad Mothers: Infertility and the Maternal Instinct', in Molly Ladd-Taylor and Lauri Umansky, *'Bad' Mothers: The Politics of Blame in Twentieth-Century America* (New York: NYU Press, 1998) 198–219.

Mehnert, Thomas., Krauss, Herbert H., Nadler, Rosemary., Boyd, Mary., 'Correlates of Life Satisfaction in Those with Disabling Conditions', *Rehabilitative Psychology*, 35/1 (1990) 3–17.

Mill, John Stuart, *Principles of Political Economy* (London: Longmans, Green & Co., 1904).

Missner, Marshall, 'Why Have Children?', *The International Journal of Applied Philosophy*, 3/4 (1987) 1–13.

Montesquieu, *Persian Letters,* trans. John Davidson, 1 (London: Gibbings & Company, 1899).

Multi-Society Task Force on PVS, 'Medical Aspects of the Persistent Vegetative State', *New England Journal of Medicine,* 330/21 (1994) 1499–508.

Myers, David G., and Diener, Ed, 'The Pursuit of Happiness', *Scientific American,* 274/5 (1996) 70–2.

Nash, Ogden, *Family Reunion* (London: J. M. Dent & Sons Ltd, 1951).

Nozick, Robert, *Anarchy, State and Utopia* (Oxford: Blackwell, 1974).

Parfit, Derek, *Reasons and Persons* (Oxford: Clarendon Press, 1984).

Pence, Gregory E., *Classic Cases in Medical Ethics,* 2nd edn. (New York, McGraw-Hill, 1995).

People and Planet, <http://www.peopleandplanet.net> (accessed 5 October 2004).

Pitcher, George, 'The Misfortunes of the Dead', *American Philosophical Quarterly,* 21/2 (1984) 183–8.

Porter, Eleanor H., *Pollyanna,* (London: George G. Harrap & Co. 1927).

Rawls, John, 'Justice as Fairness: Political not Metaphysical', *Philosophy and Public Affairs,* 14/3 (1985) 223–51.

Rees, Martin, *Our Final Hour: A Scientist's Warning* (New York: Basic Books, 2003).

Regan, Tom, 'Feinberg on What Sorts of Beings Can Have Rights?', *Southern Journal of Philosophy,* 14 (1976) 485–98.

Reuters, 'Brace yerself Sheila, it's your patriotic duty to breed', *Cape Times,* Thursday 13 May 2004, 1.

Richards, Norvin, 'Is Humility a Virtue?', *American Philosophical Quarterly,* 25/3 (1988) 253–9.

Robertson, John, *Children of Choice* (Princeton: Princeton University Press, 1994).

Rummel, R. J., *Death by Government* (New Brunswick, Transaction Publishers, 1994).

Santayana, George, *Reason in Religion* (vol. iii of *The Life of Reason*) (New York: Charles Scribner's Sons, 1922).

Schopenhauer, Arthur, 'On the Sufferings of the World', in *Complete Essays of Schopenhauer,* trans. T. Bailey Saunders (New York: Willey Book Company, 1942).

—— *The World as Will and Representation,* trans. E. F. J. Payne (New York: Dover Publications, 1966).

Schwartz, Pedro, *The New Political Economy of J.S. Mill* (London: Weiden-feld & Nicolson, 1972).

Shiffrin, Seana Valentine, 'Wrongful Life, Procreative Responsibility, and the Significance of Harm', *Legal Theory*, 5 (1999) 117–48.

Singer, Peter, Kuhse, Helga, Buckle, Stephen, Dawson, Karen, and Kasimba, Pascal, (eds.) *Embryo Experimentation* (Cambridge: Cambridge University Press, 1990).

Singer, Peter, *Practical Ethics* 2nd edn. (Cambridge: Cambridge University Press, 1993).

Smilansky, Saul, 'Is There a Moral Obligation to Have Children?', *Journal of Applied Philosophy*, 12/1 (1995) 41–53.

Sophocles, 'Oedipus at Colonus'.

Steinbock, Bonnie, *Life Before Birth* (New York: Oxford University Press, 1992) 14–24.

Suh, Eunkook., Diener, Ed, and Fujita, Frank, 'Events and Subjective Well-Being: Only Recent Events Matter', *Journal of Personality and Social Psychology*, 70/5 (1996) 1091–102.

Suits, David B., 'Why death is not bad for the one who died', *American Philosophical Quarterly*, 38/1 (2001) 69–84.

Tännsjö, Torbjörn, *Hedonistic Utilitarianism* (Edinburgh: Edinburgh University Press, 1998).

—— 'Doom Soon?', *Inquiry*, 40/2 (1997) 250–1.

Taylor, Paul W., *Respect for Nature* (Princeton: Princeton University Press, 1986).

Taylor, Shelley E., *Positive Illusions: Creative Self-Deception and the Healthy Mind* (New York: Basic Books, 1989).

—— and Brown, Jonathon D., 'Illusion and Well-Being: A Social Psychological Perspective on Mental Health', *Psychological Bulletin*, 103/2 (1998) 193–210.

Tennyson, Alfred Lord, 'In Memoriam'.

Thompson, Janna, 'A Refutation of Environmental Ethics', *Environmental Ethics*, 12/2 (1990) 147–60.

Tiger, Lionel, *Optimism: The Biology of Hope* (New York: Simon & Schuster, 1979).

Tooley, Michael, 'Abortion and Infanticide', *Philosophy and Public Affairs*, 2/1 (1972) 37–65.

Toubia, Nahid, 'Female Circumcision as a Public Health Issue', *New England Journal of Medicine*, 331/11 (1994) 712–16.

Vetter, Hermann, 'Utilitarianism and New Generations', *Mind*, 80/318 (1971) 301–2.

Voltaire, *Candide*, (London: Penguin Books, 1997).

Waller, Bruce N., 'The Sad Truth: Optimism, Pessimism and Pragmatism', *Ratio,* new series, 16 (2003) 189–97.

Wasserman, David, 'Is Every Birth Wrongful? Is Any Birth Morally Required?', DeCamp Bioethics Lecture, Princeton, 25 February 2004, unpublished manuscript.

Watts, Jonathan, 'Japan opens dating agency to improve birth rate', *The Lancet*, 360 (2002) 1755.

Weinberg, Rivka, 'Procreative Justice: A Contractualist Account', *Public Affairs Quarterly*, 16/4 (2002) 405–25.

Weinstein, Neil D., 'Unrealistic Optimism about Future Life Events', *Journal of Personality and Social Psychology*, 39/5 (1980) 806–20.

—— 'Why it Won't Happen to Me: Perceptions of Risk Factors and Susceptibility', *Health Psychology*, 3/5 (1984) 431–57.

Williams, Bernard, 'The Makropulos Case: Reflections on the Tedium of Immortality' in *Problems of the Self* (Cambridge: Cambridge University Press, 1973).

—— 'Resenting one's own existence' in *Making Sense of Humanity* (Cambridge: Cambridge University Press, 1995).

Wood, Joanne V., 'What is Social Comparison and How Should We Study it?', *Personality and Social Psychology Bulletin*, 22/5 (1996) 520–37.

World Heath Organization, *World Report on Violence and Health* (Geneva: WHO, 2002).

Yerxa, Elizabeth J., and Baum, Susan, 'Engagement in Daily Occupations and Life-Satisfaction Among People with Spinal Cord Injuries', *The Occupational Therapy Journal of Research*, 6/5 (1986) 271–83.

Index

on compensated and
uncompensated suffering 63 n.
5
on harm 21 n. 9
origin view 7 n. 8&9
population problems 168–74, 178–9,
185, 187, 190
psychological continuity 160
saving life just after it starts 24
see also impersonal views; mere
addition; non-identity problem;
person-affecting views,
repugnant conclusion; Theory
X
person-affecting views 169, 173, 186–90,
192
pessimism 69, 76, 88–9, 208–11
pollyannaism 64–9, 72, 74, 77, 78, 83,
92, 118, 119 n., *see also* optimism
procreation 6, 93–131, 206, 211, 215
and contractarianism 180, 182
and extinction 185, 193
and religion 221
see also anti-natalism; asymmetry of
duties; right to procreative
freedom
preference not to have existed 27–8,
152–5, 219
see also regretting one's existence
present-life case 22–27, 121, 212; *see also*
life (not) worth continuing
pro-natalism 8–13, 205
see also anti-natalism
pure benefit 50–54

quality of life 61–101, 118–20,
future 151, 156
Jeremiah and Job 222
and population 170–78, 182–93
relevance to death 214, 216, 218
See also disability; life (not) worth
continuing; life (not) worth
starting; life (not) worth living

Rawls, John 178, 180, 181
reductio ad absurdum 33 n. 24, 181,
204–7
Regan, Tom 138–9, 143 n.
regretting one's existence 57–9, 61,
99–100, 102, 210, 211

see also Allen, Woody; Jeremiah; Job;
preference not to have existed
reproduction, *see* artificial
reproduction; assisted
reproduction; anti-natalism;
procreation
reproductive freedom, *see* right to
procreative freedom
repugnant conclusion 171, 173–8, 182
right:
not to be created 53–4, 190–93
to abortion 162
to citizenship 12
to continued life 148–9; *see also*
interests in continued existence
to do wrong 103
to immigrate 12
to procreative freedom 12, 102–113,
122, 128, 162
violation of a 53, 150

Schopenhauer, Arthur 60, 76–7, 81 n.
39, 89, 163
sentience 2, 209, 223, 224
sexual ethics 125–7, 221
Shammai 222–3
Shiffrin, Seana 49–54, 100
S(ick) and H(ealthy), analogy of 42–3,
47, 49
Singapore 10
Singer, Peter 33 n. 24, 202
social comparison, *see* comparison,
social
Stoics 81
sub specie aeternitatis 81–6, 199
sub specie humanitatis 81–6
suicide 69, 91–2, 211–21

Tännsjö, Torbjörn 171 n.
Taylor, Paul W. 137–40
Theory X 169–70, 172–80
Tooley, Michael 148–50
treadmill of desires 75–7

utilitarianism 36–7, 88, 189, 202

Voltaire 92, 219

Weinberg, Rivka 6 n. 6, 179, 180 n. 36
wrongful life 22 n. 12, 23 n. 14, 113–4,
122–4

Printed and bound by CPI Group (UK) Ltd, Croydon, CR0 4YY